The Human Effect in Medicine

Theory, research and practice

Michael Dixon

General Practitioner, Devon
Research Fellow, University of Exet~
Chair, NHS Alli~

and

Kieran Swee~~~~

General Practitioner, Devon
Lecturer in General Practice,
Postgraduate Medical School,
University of Exeter

Foreword by

Sir Denis Pereira Gray

Professor of General Practice,
University of Exeter
President, Royal College of General Practitioners

Radcliffe Medical Press

Radcliffe Medical Press
18 Marcham Road, Abingdon, Oxon OX14 1AA

British Library Cataloguing in Publication Data

A catalogue record for this book is available from the British Library.

ISBN 1 85775 369 0

Typeset by Joshua Associates Ltd., Oxford
Printed and bound by TJ International Ltd., Padstow, Cornwall

Contents

Foreword

Pendulums swing in most fields of life, and medicine and general practice are no exceptions. At the mid-point of the twentieth century, when the College of General Practitioners was founded in 1952, the human side of medicine was well understood and implicitly accepted by most working practitioners. The brilliantly constructed motto of the College, *'Cum Scientia Caritas'* ('Care with science'), was adopted by the College in 1957 and summarises masterly the role of the clinical generalist. Importantly, it put the care component first.

Nineteen years later, Professor Avedis Donabedian in the USA, re-stated this duo using as his terms 'technical competence' and 'interpersonal factors'.[1] As the century progressed, the personal aspects came second.

In the second half of the century came a string of intellectual contributions, which greatly influenced thought in general practice. Logan and Cushion showed the importance of practical epidemiology in general practice, Illich challenged the whole basis of the doctor's role and McKeown emphasised the importance of environmental factors in affecting health.[2–4]

Later still, from York, a new emphasis on cost effectiveness such as 'Quality Adjusted Life Years' (QUALYs) and 'Evidence-based Medicine' (EBM).[5,6] Each of these illuminated the nature of the discipline and enriched GPs' understanding of their role. But each of these came at a price – that the impersonal was being repeatedly valued at the expense of the personal.

Measurable organisational changes such as larger partnerships, greater teams and more extensive cover arrangements, also contributed to this. Fundholding and PCGs both emphasised the group versus the individual. Thus, personal aspects of the discipline slowly and gradually came under threat.

It is likely that historians will see Sackett's EBM movement as the trigger. Its tidy intellectual logic, and apparently simple case, challenging doctors, especially personal doctors, to review again the core meaning of medicine. EBM may prove to have been the point when the pendulum of thought started to swing back again from the impersonal aspects of general practice medicine towards the personal. Two recent RCGP William Pickles Lectures have been particularly influential.[7,8]

The current generation of GPs has started to rise to this task. *The Human Effect in Medicine* comes from this stable, showing that a new generation of theorists is emerging from the book's authors[9,10] and others.[11–17]

This book uses old words like 'suffering' and 'healing' in new ways, illuminating old theories with new evidence. The writing packs punch: 'it now seems that *Caritas* means not just care, but cure'. That sentence is the summary of this text, which is a valuable addition to the literature of medicine.

Professor Sir Denis Pereira Gray
OBE FRCP PRCGP FMedSci
January 2000

References

1   Donabedian A (1979) The quality of medical care: a concept in search of a definition. First Ward Darley Lecture. *J Fam Prac.* **9**: 277–84.

2   Logan WPD, Cushion AA (1958) *Morbidity Statistics from General Practice. Volumes 1 and 2.* HMSO, London.

3   Illich I (1974) *Medical Nemesis.* Calder and Boyars, London.

4   McKeown T (1976) *The Role of Medicine: dream, mirage or nemesis?* Rock Carling Lecture. Nuffield Provincial Hospitals Trust, London.

5   Drummond MF, Maynard A (eds) (1993) *Purchasing and Providing Cost-effective Health Care.* Churchill Livingstone, Edinburgh.

6   Sackett DL, Richardson WS, Rosenberg W, Haynes RB (1997) *Evidence Based Medicine: how to teach and practise EBM.* Churchill Livingstone, Edinburgh.

7   McWhinney IR (1996) The importance of being different. William Pickles Lecture. *Br J Gen Prac.* **46**: 433–6.

8 Heath I (1999) Uncertain clarity: contradiction, meaning, and hope. William Pickles Lecture. *Br J Gen Prac.* **49:** 651–7.

9 Sweeney KG, MacAuley J, Pereira Gray D (1998) Personal significance: the third dimension. *Lancet.* **351:** 134–6.

10 Dixon DM, Sweeney KG, Pereira Gray DJ (1999) The physician healer: ancient magic or modern science? *Br J Gen Prac.* **49:** 309–12.

11 Pew Fetzer Task Force on Advancing Psychosocial Health Education (1994) *Relationship-centered Care.* Pew Fetzer, California.

12 Baker R, Streatfield J (1995) What type of general practice do patients prefer? Exploration of practice characteristics influencing patient satisfaction. *J R Coll Gen Practitioner.* **45:** 654–9.

13 Heath I (1995) *The Mystery of General Practice.* The Nuffield Provincial Hospitals Trust, London.

14 Greenhalgh T, Hurwitz B (eds) (1998) *Narrative Based Medicine: dialogue and discourse in clinical practice.* BMJ Publishing, London.

15 Gulbrandsen P, Fugelli P, Sandvik L, Hjortdahl P (1998) Influence of social problems on management in general practice: multi-practice questionnaire survey. *BMJ.* **317:** 28–32.

16 Howie JGR, Heaney DJ, Maxwell M (1997) *Measuring Quality in General Practice. Occasional Paper 75.* RCGP, Exeter.

17 Toon PD (1999) *Towards a Philosophy of General Practice: a study of the virtuous practitioner. Occasional Paper 78.* RCGP, London.

Preface

Our primary aim was to write a book for general practitioners. We hope nevertheless that it will be of use and interest to all doctors, nurses, health managers, policy makers and even the patients themselves. That is because the human effect is as relevant to them as it is to genereal practitioners. This book describes how modern medicine is failing to deliver and why a more human approach is required. It reviews the vast weight of evidence on the effectiveness of the human effect and finally tries to use some of this evidence in order to describe how we can use the human effect in our everyday practice. The authors make no apology for providing references at every twist and turn of this narrative as we are keen that these ideas should not be dismissed as the ramblings of two medical dinosaurs.

Michael Dixon
Kieran Sweeney
January 2000

Acknowledgements

There is little new under the sun and many of the thoughts in this book started elsewhere. Writers such as Herbert Benson in the USA and Ian McWhinney in Canada have both written about the need for a holistic approach in medicine and greatly influenced our thinking. On this side of the Atlantic, Michael Balint has been an important authority as have Annie Mitchell and Maggie McCormack, clinical psychologists at Exeter University, who have studied these effects in complementary medicine. For one of us (MD) personal contact with complementary practitioners, who are experts in the human effect, has been a major influence; in particular, Gill White, who works in his practice.

Thanks are also to David Greaves of the Institute of Philosophy and Health Care at the University of Swansea and also to Peter Toon, whose recent contributions to the philosophy of general practice have been deeply illuminating. Professor Sir Denis Pereira Gray has been a constant supporter of our work and an invaluable source of general advice and research evidence from general practice. His help would not have been possible without the secretarial help of Annie Hills. We would also like to thank other colleagues who are part of the Exeter team that is working on the therapeutic relationship – Dr Martin Marshall, Phil Evans, Nick Bradley and Sindy Banga.

On a personal level, thanks are due to both our families. MD would like to thank his wife Joanna for her patience and support. His lucky fortune is to receive ample helpings of the human effect on a daily basis not only from her but also from his children Finn, May and Liberty. Also his parents, Hazel and Tony, who hand it out effortlessly to everyone around them.

KS would like to thank his wife Barbara, and Patrick, Michael, Kieran and Louise, his four children, for putting up with his absences as this book was in preparation.

Penultimate thanks to Heidi Allen and Gillian Nineham of Radcliffe Medical Press, who have been always encouraging and admirably patient with our slow progress on this project. Last but not least, Christine Quinn, MD's secretary, who has once again done the impossible and singlehandedly produced a book from tapes that were invariably produced on the hoof and with background noises that must have driven her to distraction. All of which is not to forget our patients, who provided the practical experience, proof and inspiration for this work.

To James Sweeney who would have supported the ideas behind this book and to Patrick Dixon who practised them on a daily basis.

CHAPTER ONE

Introduction

Michael Dixon

The title of this book may seem presumptuous. It is meant to be. Our intention is to challenge the dogma of modern technological medicine that ignores both the therapeutic effect of the doctor and the self-healing powers of the patient. This was an understandable dogma, when doctors first found themselves armed with effective medicines and procedures, to which they had never previously had access. It was acceptable too, when the National Health Service (NHS) could afford all new medications and procedures and when each brought a significant cost benefit. Those times are over.

Western medicine is now facing a crisis. Modern technology, its very life blood, is failing to deliver the goods. This goes deeper than our inability to cure a whole range of common and serious diseases. Further than the truth that it is often used inappropriately, for instance, in the elderly or the unhappy where psychological or environmental factors are frequently more relevant than the medicine itself. Nor is it simply a question that we are eroding our natural knowledge and ability to heal ourselves by using modern medicines where simple remedies or change of lifestyle might suffice or indeed where the illness is self-limiting anyway. The main problem, the bottom line, is that we can no longer afford modern technology. It is likely to become increasingly unavailable within the NHS and thus become increasingly irrelevant to the health of the majority. The technology that we do have will continue to be rationed through long waiting lists, which are themselves a cause of morbidity and may nullify any beneficial effects when the patient finally receives it.

Magnetic resonance imaging (MRI) scans are an example. A brilliant means of being able to look at every part of the body in minute detail – yet demand far outweighs supply in the NHS. The government indirectly sets financial limits for such scans with its agenda being set by the voter and taxpayer. Highly skilled doctors order scans for their patients along evidence-based guidelines – overall more scans than the money allows for. The result is that patients may wait up to a year or 18 months in order to find out, for instance, whether their headache signifies a brain tumour, or whether numbness and pins and needles are due to multiple sclerosis. Thus patients wait anxiously for an investigation that turns out to be normal in the majority and for symptoms that were probably dealt with as (if not more) adequately before the technology was available. It is only one example but it raises the question of whether we should end-lessly fight disease by throwing technology at it, especially when we are unable to deliver that technology without frustrating and stressful delays. Perhaps we should concentrate more on main-taining health and resistance to disease in the first place?

As we begin to realise the limits of our technology as health professionals, our patients are concerned that modern medicine offers little else. Many complain about the impersonality of modern general practice, which might require them to see one of many doctors in a busy health centre and be visited at night by doctors whom they have never met before. Indeed according to a recent *Which?* report, general practitioners (GPs) thought it was more important to offer technically correct medicine in a centre with many associated health services, while all the patient appeared to be looking for was someone who would give them time, understand them and reassure them. The 'personal touch' has somehow been lost in the emphasis on providing evidence-based medicine, yet research on the placebo effect suggests that this may be by far the most effective and generalisable medicine that we have. Instead of developing our skills in achieving better placebo effects, we decry it as a nuisance factor, which messes up our clinical trials on new drugs and procedures. For many years, it seems, we have simply missed the plot.

Double-blind, placebo-controlled trials show an average placebo effect of around 30%. But these '*in vitro*' results have little bearing on what almost certainly happens in the average general practice consultation '*in vivo*'. It is one thing for a patient to be told that he or she may or may not have active medication. Quite another for a very motivated patient to take on a treatment that both he or she and their GP feel to be effective and which fits within a whole theoretical and cultural framework. The extent of this effect will vary according to the doctor, patient and the condition, however, '*in vivo*' studies of treatments that are now discredited but were once regarded as mainstream showed a 50–70% cure rate in their time. It is not just a question of feeling better but of actually being better as evidenced by the healing rate of stomach ulcers (proven on endoscopy), which is around 45% for patients given a placebo in a double-blind, placebo-controlled trial. Thus the placebo or therapeutic effect depends to a large degree on the extent to which the doctor has the skills or the motivation to produce maximum impact. Yet this is an area that medical teaching on evidence-based medicine has ignored completely.

It is odd that modern medicine, which increasingly emphasises evidence, has failed to look at the possibility of exploiting this major effect as a means of not only making patients better but also saving on expensive modern medicines and techniques. For instance, if we could remove only 10% of patients from the conventional diagnostic, referral and treatment pathway or amplify the effects of treatment by only 10% for patients that did enter such a pathway, this would have major financial implications for the health service. Not least it would allow modern technology to be provided rapidly for those who did need it.

The placebo effect is about enabling patients to rediscover their self-healing powers. This is the basis of the 'New medicine' but it is in fact a very old medicine – a rediscovery. Hippocrates saw the role of the doctor as that of 'medical attendant to the patient's own self-healing powers'. So the 'new medicine' is really a re-description of this role in the light of modern evidence on how we can optimise our role in catalysing the self-healing powers of our patients. As we shall see, it is a role that goes far beyond simply telling patients that they must pull their socks up and look after themselves. Such advice is hardly helpful to the demoralised or those who have poor self-esteem (i.e. the majority of our long-term patients). For some patients, we will be able to maximise the placebo effect in each consultation. For others, it will be a process that requires great adaptiveness, which could involve supporting and nurturing patients at a low ebb, while enabling those same patients to develop their own role in self-treatment as they become stronger.

If patients can heal themselves (what else is happening in a self-limiting medical illness?) and if doctors are able to flick the switch that turns these powers on – then it makes little sense to distinguish between mind and body. Nor would it be right to over-professionalise the doctor's role in this process. Our possession of powerful healing tools (in the western medical tradition) has provided us with powerful healing powers (in a sense of being able to catalyse the patient's own self-healing). Nevertheless, other therapists, particularly complementary therapists and nurses, are particularly good at this and we should be encouraging whole communities to realise the similar powers that each individual can potentially exert on another. It seems highly likely that the actual degree of such self-healing within a community might depend on its 'social capital' and that the cohesiveness, goodwill and morale of a community might be major factors.

Primary care groups and trusts represent a threat and an opportunity for the physician healer. A threat, that is if we limit ourselves to the limited evidence base, ignore the issues raised in this book and concentrate on symptoms, diseases and health services rather than health. Ideally, however, they should represent an opportunity as the 'holistic' message of the 'new medicine' fits nicely within the 'new NHS' with its emphasis on local communities and looking at health in a wider context than simply health services. This allows health professionals to focus on the overall health of their communities as a means of not only improving health, but also demand managing access to scarce technology. An holistic view of the patient in the surgery and an holistic view of the health of the local population – holistic solutions to problems that have not been solved previously by fragmented answers. They could provide a powerful antidote to the limitations both of our individual therapeutic role and the role of health services in general. Balint echoed this vision in 1957 describing his version of general practice in Utopia. 'The general practitioner will no longer be able to disappear behind the strong and impenetrable facade of a bored, overworked but not very responsible dispenser of drugs and writer of innumerable letters, certificates and requests for examinations; instead he will have to shoulder the privilege of undivided responsibility for peoples' health and wellbeing, and partly for their future happiness'.

Although our explicit aim should be to improve the health of patients and their ability to withstand disease, 'new medicine' is not simply about patients. It should provide a new balance in the consultation for doctors at a time when recruitment in general practice is becoming difficult and where the trust between doctor and patient seems to be breaking down. A new balance between Jung's 'animus', which is the modern way of treating illness and the 'anima, which is the level upon which most patients experience their disease and are looking for help. A new balance between evidence and philosophy and between professional responsibility and self-care. If we can restore the self-healing processes of the patient then the result could be doctors who are happy in their work and patients who are happy with themselves and with their doctors.

Many doctors reading this book will exclaim: 'Well I am doing that already!' For those doctors, the message is that modern research is supporting their approach, that it is beginning to value what they are doing and that it is starting to look at how we might even do it better. For the less converted, ask yourself a few questions: Do you get fed up with patients, who you can't make better or who won't help themselves? Do you feel that your surgeries are full of illnesses that really do not require your professional opinion? Do you think that there is more to the health of your patients than their presenting symptoms? Do you come across a number of patients whom you can neither diagnose nor treat successfully? Do you sometimes feel that you are battering your head against a brick wall and see the patient as the enemy? Do you dread the next patient and do you find it increasingly difficult to either like or sympathise with them? Does your work drain and exhaust you? If the answer to any of these questions is yes then perhaps you should read on. Not because this will change your practice with each and every patient, it may, but to arm you with a perceptual shift that could make your work more satisfying.

This book is about a vision. A vision that GPs and patients will recognise and regain their therapeutic potential. A vision that body will meet mind, that West will meet East and that doctor will meet patient in a more fulfilling encounter. It is a vision that we describe from a medical point of view as it would be presumptuous to go beyond our field of experience, although the principle should apply to all caring professions. This book, however, is not just about ideas. It is also a concerted attempt to analyse those aspects of the GP's role that add to his/her therapeutic potential. A detailed prescription, it cannot be, partly because of the early state of the art and partly because exact instructions might lead to a form of grotesque mimicry, which can only detract from the intuition and empathy of the individual GP, which is essential to his/her role as a therapist. So do not ask for too much detailed information or concrete evidence – that is an essential part of modern medicine but not necessarily that of becoming a successful doctor/healer. All that we can offer are a few tips based on the experiences and evidence of others. The main aim of this book is to provide a shift in perspective on what we can achieve as doctors. To welcome the dawn of a new medicine.

PART ONE

The philosophy and history of medical practice: a review

Kieran Sweeney

CHAPTER TWO

Challenging the current therapeutic perspective

The hegemony of science in medicine is under serious threat.[1,2] Its demise can be dated from the publication in 1992 of the manifesto of the Evidence Based Medicine Working Group,[3] which challenged the profession over its failure to apply, vigorously and consistently, the principles of biomedicine, predicated as it is on scientific positivism and a linear explanatory model. The ensuing rise to power of the evidence-based medicine (EBM) movement was swift and spectacular, aided in no small part by the support of politicians attracted by its perceived clarity and appealing simplicity. Information was king, counting became the currency of conclusion. EBM became the new deity, espoused by clinicians, worshiped by managers and demanded by politicians.

One of the effects of the spectacular rise of EBM to its central position in the delivery of healthcare in the NHS was to galvanise those who remained cautious or sceptical about its claims to improve care simply through the applications of its principle. Commentaries from general practices began to emerge, and a definitive counter statement was set out in the form of a seminal text published through the Nuffield Hospitals Provincial Trust.[4,5] Heath's *Mystery of General Practice* espoused a much wider view of the role of the doctor in healthcare. The author identified three general responsibilities for the doctor: interpreting a patient's story, acting at the interface between health and disease, and guarding against over-medicalisation. Even its language stood in sharp contrast to the robust numeracy of the EBM publications.

The principal success of the EBM movement has been to clarify and refine their view of the nature of clinical practice into three central characteristics.[6] It is predicated on science, processed by rational thinking and perceived, as a function of these two, to have clear outcomes; clarity, or rather perceived clarity, is the third characteristic.

That these are the central features of contemporary medical practice cannot seriously be doubted. The first of these, the scientific basis of biomedicine is beyond argument. As practitioners we espouse a positivist approach to our thinking, we hold an ontological concept of disease, which views disease in technical and reductionist terms. We are followers of enlightenment thought – disciples of Descartes. The system of clinical practice, which this philosophy supports, regards itself as evolving and progressive, ultimately capable of resolving as yet unsolved problems. It is a system that regards itself as having a constant capacity for improvement, an almost irresistible power to solve puzzles and explain everything.

The rationality of contemporary clinical practice has Cartesian origins, which have been explicitly restated by the leading exponent of the EBM movement.[7] In his classic text, *Clinical Epidemiology*, Professor David Sackett[6] writes, 'in all this, the assumption is that medicine is rational and so are you'. In this book, we shall argue that neither of these propositions can be supported unequivocally: medicine is not exclusively logical and neither are its practitioners.

The clarion call to the perceived clarity of contemporary clinical practice is epitomised by the stream of documents currently being distributed by the Department of Health to support the emergence of primary care groups (PCGs) as the central focus of the reorganisation of the NHS. In particular the document entitled *First Class Service* is presented with a concealed, but firm, conviction that there is certainty in clinical practice, which is just not getting through to the right people in the right way or at the right time; if it did care would be more effective.[8] These documents represent the politicisation of EBM.

In this chapter we question the assumptions that support these three central features of contemporary clinical practice. We argue that there is no absolute universal notion of science, either in philosophical or in historical terms, which should afford a position of unassailable centrality in clinical practice. We accept that the practice and understanding of medicine demands in part a rational appreciation and cognitive evaluation of information. But it goes beyond that to involve inextricably the *self*, both the practitioner's self and the patient's self. We argue that the clarity so appealing to politicians is illusory and disingenuous, based on an inadequate explanatory model that is predicated on linear thinking, now recognised to be inappropriate for explaining the complexities and constantly evolving nature of the human condition.[9] The metaphysics of health and disease cannot be explained simply by a series of causes and effects.

The nature of science in medical practice

The contemporary notion of science in medicine is a fairly recent acquisition.[2] As clinical practitioners, doctors embrace a positivist, rationalist philosophy of medicine, they support an ontological view of disease and they regard areas of medical ignorance simply as unsolved puzzles.

This approach was not recognised before 1800 and really gained central recognition with the establishment only as part of the Medical Act, 1858, of the General Medical Council (GMC). More than anything, it was this act which set the central tenets of the contemporary medical model in blocks of political stone. The act defined a particular system of training and of registration, which demarcated the essence of clinical practice, gave its practitioners – only those within the system of registration – rights above all over practitioners who were then relegated to a secondary 'alternative' category. For the first time the pivotal position of medical practitioners in the system of healthcare was assured.

The question then arises, does the place of science as the basis for this medical model justify itself in the way that is promoted by the medical profession, encouraged by civil servants and currently accepted by society?

The common sense view of science holds that scientific knowledge is real because it is based on what we can hear, see and touch. It is held to be reliable because it is objective, a term that importantly implies that it is value neutral. Scientific knowledge and laws are derived from dispassionate serial observation, conducted in controlled experimental environments. This common sense view of science in medicine really derives from the Enlightenment, developed in the seventeenth century, and emerging principally from the work of Descartes, Bacon and Newton. However, Chalmers,[10] among others, describes this view of science as naive, quite mistaken and dangerously misleading.

The common sense view of science described above is an inductivist view. Inductivists argue that, providing initial conditions are observed, universal laws can be generated from a finite list of single observations. Thus, scientific knowledge is built up serially from these observations, which ultimately allow the observer to generalise about the outcome of the observation. For many years this was the basis of medical undergraduate teaching; diagnosis was constructed from a series of observations, measurements and tests which could provide the overall solution or diagnosis, using an inductive process. And in the physical sciences, inductivist thinking works well. The eclipse of the sun on 11 August 1999 was predicted accurately on the basis of induction following a series of observations.

This portrayal of the philosophy underpinning the currently accepted notion of science in medical practice is not simply of esoteric, arcane interest. Reflect for a moment on what this approach is arguing as a general principle. The inductivist approach argues that the process of induction has worked in a series of circumstances A, circumstances B, C and so on; because the principle has worked in a finite series of circumstances, the argument proceeds, then the principle of induction works. But this is of course a circular argument, one cannot use induction to prove induction. A second weakness of the inductivist argument derives from the view that all observational statements presuppose theory. Consider the frustration of the night-time riser, who, stumbling in the dark reaches out for the light, only to exclaim 'dash, the bulb has gone'. Even this simple statement assumes that there is a substance, presumably electricity, which can be conveyed in an object (a lamp), the nature of which would allow for illumination through the conversion of electrical energy to a mixture of heat and light, and that the result will render the riser's journey more simple, an expectation which is revealed by the frustration with which the remark is delivered.

As the theoretical predicates which inform an observation become more complex, so the perceptions flowing from an observation become more detailed. Michael Polanyi,[11] in his seminal book *Personal Knowledge*, gives the example of how a medical student's perceptions of an X-ray become more detailed and informed as he learns more about the theory of diagnostic radiology. Polanyi writes,

> 'At first the student is completely puzzled by the x-ray. He can see in the x-ray picture of a chest only the shadows of the heart and ribs, with a few spidery blotches between them. The experts seem to be romancing about figments of their imagination; he can see nothing that they are talking about. Then as he goes on listening for a few weeks, looking carefully at ever new pictures of different cases, a tentative understanding will dawn on him; he will gradually forget about the ribs and begin to see the lungs. And eventually, if he perseveres intelligently, a rich panorama of significant details will be revealed to him; of physiological variations, pathological changes, of scars, of chronic infection and signs of acute disease. He has entered a New World. He still sees only a fraction of what the experts can see but the pictures are definitely making sense now and so do most of the comments made on them.'

Clearly, this inductivist view of science could not withstand philosophical critique: it begged modification. Karl Popper tried to reform this absolute view of science by constructing the position of falsificationism.[12] Falsificationists accept the circularity of the inductivist view of science, and they accept that observations are theory dependent also; they abandon any claim that general theories can be established by serial observations. What Popper and the falsificationists argue is that scientific theories are in fact speculative guesses, which are set out in the scientific community to be ruthlessly assessed and tested. Those that survive attempts at falsification are robust, others go by the wayside. Great prestige is accorded to theories that are speculated on the basis of current knowledge, but which cannot be tested or falsified for many years, and when they are so tested withstand the attempt. One example of this is the projection from Einstein's theory of relativity.

Chalmers[10] recounts how Popper criticised the notion of absolutism in science:

> *'The empirical basis for objective science has nothing absolute about it, science does not rest upon a solid bed rock. The bold structures of its theories rise as it were above a swamp. It is like a building erected on piles. The piles are driven down from above into the swamp but not down to any natural or given base. If we stop driving the piles deeper it is not because we have reached any firm ground. We simply stop when we are satisfied. The piles are firm enough to carry the structure at least for the time being.'*[12]

But even this modified Popperian position is not beyond reproach. The observational statements which Popper advocates should be used as the mechanism of assessment for a scientific theory are themselves fallible, in as much as they are as theory dependent as the observations they are trying to falsify.

If one criticises successive philosophical approaches to thinking in science in this way one cannot leave a void where the only conclusion is that there is no justification for any particular theory of science. Chalmers[10] settles for the position of *unrepresentative realism*, arguing that the physical world *is* such that the physical theories deriving from, for example, Einstein are applicable to it, and do explain the world to some degree. His position is *unrepresentative* because it does not assume that physical theories describe actual entities in the world, for example, sound waves or magnetic fields, in a way that corresponds to ordinary common sense sensory input. His notion is, however, *realist* because it does accept that theories are applicable to the world both inside and outside experimental situations, and that these theories do associate events beyond simply observing connections in experimental situations.

What is the point of evaluating the notion of science in medicine from this esoteric philosophical point of view? There are two important reasons. First, the limitations of inductivist-ism, observational statements and the vulnerability of falsifica-tionism support the view that there is no timeless or universal concept of science or the scientific method which demands intellectual hegemony. As Chalmers[10] argues 'we cannot legiti-mately except or exclude an item of knowledge simply because it does not conform to our view of science'. Thus, the firm conviction held throughout the whole of the twentieth century that the strength of medical practice has its very basis in science, is seen to be unsupportable at its very philosophical origins.

Secondly, and perhaps more importantly, this analysis raises the point that the view of science currently espoused by practitioners, demanded by managers and applauded by politi-cians has devalued an intellectual standpoint into an ideology. When Curtis Bok advocated disseminating 'the benefits of science for all doctors and patients' he was not supporting an intellectually celibate view – in fact he was arguing against comprehensive personal health insurance in the US (quoted in Porter[13]). More recently, in *First Class Service*, the Secretary of State for Health[8] clearly supported this view of science, deeming it to be capable of producing 'evidence which can promote clear guidelines for which treatments are best for which patients'. Given the uniqueness of the individual illness experience and the enormous pitfalls in transferring scientific evidence into individual clinical practice (a matter which will be discussed later in the book), this can be regarded as an almost unknowable proposition. Thus, not only is the notion of science fallible in itself, but its use as an ideology in politics both within and outside the medical profession currently constitutes a serious cause for concern. Medicine, alongside any of the other science, cannot claim to have an unassailable view of how the world works.

References

1   Evans M, Sweeney KG (1998) *The Human Side of Medicine*. Royal College of General Practitioners, London.

2 Greaves D (1996) *Mystery in Western Medicine.* Ashgate Publishing Limited, Aldershot, UK.

3 Evidence Based Medicine Working Group (1992) Evidence based medicine: a new approach to teaching the practice of medicine. *JAMA* **268**: 2420–5.

4 Sweeney KG (1996) Evidence and uncertainty. In: M Marinker (ed.) *Sense and Sensibility in Health Care.* BMJ Publishing, London.

5 Heath I (1995) *The Mystery of General Practice.* Nuffield Hospitals Provincial Trust, London.

6 Sackett DL, Haynes RB, Tugwell P (1985) *Clinical Epidemiology: a basic science for clinical medicine.* Little Brown, Boston.

7 Russell B (1961) *The History of Western Philosophy.* Unwin Paperbacks, London.

8 Secretary of State for Health (1998) *A First Class Service.* Department of Health, London.

9 Funcowicz S, Ravetz JR (1994) Emergent complex systems. *Futures* **26**: 568–82.

10 Chalmers AF (1978) *What is This Thing Called Science?* University of Queensland Press, St Lucia, Queensland.

11 Polanyi M (1973) *Personal Knowledge.* Routledge and Kegan Paul, London.

12 Popper C (1960) *The Logic of Scientific Discovery.* Hutchinson, London.

13 Porter R (1997) *The Greatest Benefit to Mankind.* Fontana Press, London.

CHAPTER THREE

Challenging the conventional history of clinical practice

Why does western medicine view itself in the way it does? What are the historical elements that came together to produce the traditional medical model based on the positivist conception of science which has been critiqued in Chapter One? This chapter reviews the conventional analysis of the history of medicine and offers the view that, just as the intellectual basis for medical thinking can be challenged, so too can the historical basis for clinical practice.

Conventionally, the historical view of medicine starts in ancient Greece with the various texts collected under the names of Hippocrates and Plato, whose writings are commonly combined in most historical analyses. Their esteemed legacy, beyond any doubt, is rationality in medicine. Hippocrates is credited with freeing science from the influence of demons and mysteries; Plato wrote that the healhy mind, body and indeed society were the consequence of the rule of reason.[1] Medicine, Plato argued, must construct and reflect a rational understanding of the workings of the human body. As a consequence of this rationality, medical thinking in ancient Greece is credited with developing the ontological notion of an illness as a specific entity, out there somewhere in the real physical sense. Moreover, the empirical approach to detailed observation, which the ancient Greeks advocated, is considered by conventional commentators of medical thinking to be a much valued legacy, exceeded only by the ethical principles which still form the basis of the oath sworn by all practising physicians.

Taking these developments in ancient Greece as the starting

point for the history of medicine, what is now referred to as the Whig view of history presents subsequent developments as part of a predetermined thread, as inevitable as it was intellectually justifiable, imbuing the knowledge and the events with a status that has only recently been challenged.[2,3]

The works of Hippocrates and the subsequent development of those ideas by Plato do not display a total agreement or an exclusive intellectual basis in reason. Dubos,[2] while accepting an almost biblical centrality for Hippocrates, argues that his importance lies with the universality, the catholicity of his message. In the writings of Hippocrates, Dubot argues 'everyone can find in them something relevant to his preoccupation'.

This view of medical history moves on into Roman times and identifies Galen as the principal influence.[4] Galen was a prolific author with almost 350 authentic titles bearing his name. He was a true medical scientist, carrying out meticulous anatomical dissection, setting up scientific experiments and, on the basis of these, formulating a view about the internal workings of the body in terms of physiological structure and function; setting the work of Hippocrates within the wider anatomo-physiological framework is considered his main achievement.[5]

The rationalist view, which pervades the Whig analysis of the history of medical thinking, is barely concealed in the period subsequent to the Roman Empire, the millennium following the year 200. One need look no further than the title the Dark Ages to sense the disdain with which this period is regarded. But not everyone shares this disdain for the period, at least as far as medicine is concerned. Greaves[3] argues forcibly that the Middle Ages represents the period of diversity in medical practice, in which a large number of variables was held to cause, explain, alter and reconcile illness and disease. Spiritual healing flourished; each organ in the body acquired a saint to whom one could pray for intercession. Benedictine monks ranked the care of the sick above all other responsibilities, and opened hospitals for sick monks and later the general public.[5] Such diversity is regarded by some commentators an asset, not a flaw, mainly because the prevailing philosophical approach during the Middle Ages accepted man's inherent inability to understand or cope with the complexities of the world. There was, Greaves argues, a prevailing sense of 'mystery'.[3]

While 1500 probably marks the end of the Dark Ages, the value-laden title of the subsequent period in history again points to the conspicuous preference for rationality and positivism in the conventional analysis of medicine. Thus, the description of Renaissance or Enlightenment clearly reveals a predeliction for that 300-year period following 1500 when the restoration of intellectual thinking based on rationality was strongly welcomed. This is without doubt the period of history that most strongly influences contemporary medical thinking, mainly through the writings of Bacon, Newton and Descartes. It was Bacon who first related the manifestations of illness in real life to the pathological changes in the morbid state in his classic *Advancement of Learning.* Newton's mechanical series of laws provided a highly desirable mechanistic set of metaphors for medical practice to use.

One of the earliest examples of the application of Newton's laws in clinical practice was Harvey's description of the circulation in 1628. Harvey was the first to describe the idea of circulation as the basis for the movement of blood – previous explanatory models were based on a poorly developed notion of ebb and flow. Harvey based this explanation on the simple, but at the time quite radical, observation that the amount of blood which flowed from the heart in an hour far exceeded the total blood volume. The contribution of Harvey's explanation of circulation cannot be underestimated. His contribution is still considered to be the basis of physiology and is utterly central to the rationalist basis of clinical medicine even today.

If Harvey is seen as the main influence on clinical practice, it is Descartes[6] who remains central to medical thinking, and its underpinning philosophy. His expression of mind–body dualism and his development of the ontological concept of disease centralised rational positivist thinking in medicine in a way that remains virtually unaltered today.

Perhaps less widely known, but equally central to the development of clinical practice, in the Enlightenment period was the contribution of Sydenham who practised in London in the second half of the seventeenth century. Sydenham was the first to systematically link individual case observations in a way that began to create a taxonomy of typicality in clinical presentation (although in doing so he could stand accused of naïve inductivism, an approach which we criticised in Chapter One). Greaves[3] offers a further insightful comment on Sydenham's contribution to clinical thinking. Sydenham's achievement derives from his meticulous approach to describing disease through disciplined observations of clinical clues and pathophysiological facts whose nature and significance could only be appreciated by a physician. Prior to that descriptions of illness were inextricably linked with the patient's own view and values concerning health and illness. Up to that point the single case history was the basic unit of education in medical practice: now there was a new medical understanding that combined theory and observation in a systematic way which only doctors could understand because of their particular expertise. In this way, Greaves argues, the nature of the relationship between the doctor and the patient was redefined.

It is during the last 200 years of the present millennium that one sees the real triumph of rationalism and scientific thinking in medicine. The nineteenth century saw the dawn of hospital medicine in Paris. Foucault identifies the Parisian clinician Bichat's work in anatomy as pivotal at this time. 'The great break in the history of Western medicine', Foucault observes, 'dates precisely from the moment clinical experience became the anatomo-clinical gaze'.[7]

Laboratory medicine then developed following the publication in 1891 of Koch's postulates. In essence, Koch proposed that a disease could be defined as being present if three elements were found: the causal agent, the pathological lesion and the clinical syndrome. Alongside Louis Pasteur, whose work describing micro-organisms and their role in diseases was equally important, Koch set the scene for the development of germ theory as a central concept in western medicine and gave rise to the entire discipline that came to be known as microbiology.[8] Medicine was moving inexorably away from the bedside, into the hospital and the laboratory. A hierarchy within medical practice would stratify itself in relationship to these locations; the seniority of the hospital-based physician above those who worked in the community and those who concerned themselves with public medicine was revealed for the first time.

The scene was now set for an expansion of science-based medicine with its positivist conceptions and reductionist techniques. In Germany, interest moved from gross anatomy to histology, biochemistry and microbiology. Concomitant developments in statistical thinking also helped the application of the scientific method giving rise to the practice of epidemiology; 1893 saw the first edition of the *International List of Causes of Death*, revisions of which are still in use today as the *International Statistical Classification of Diseases*. At last medicine had broken free from subjectivity and, maybe more importantly, the patient's perspective; scientific rationalism and its empirical applications were hailed as huge benefits, value-free and morally neutral.[3]

In summary, the conventional history of medicine, runs thus: after an early golden age of rationalism at the time of the ancient Greeks, came a lost period during the Dark Ages, followed by a welcome intellectual recovery during the Enlightenment. Encouraging developments in germ theory during the later part of the nineteenth century allowed the traditions started by Sydenham in clinical medicine, Bichat in pathology and Pasteur and Koche in microbiology to proceed apace. Subsequent developments in mathematics, statistics and investigative radiology focused the interest of practising clinicians more and more down to the scientific basis of medical practice. A full taxonomy was developing. Remaining areas of ignorance were simply puzzles waiting to be solved, not mysteries forever eluding the investigator. 'Medicine never really got anywhere until it threw metaphysics overboard' thundered Henry Mencken (presumably with some relief) in a minority medical report in 1951, 'show me a medical man who still toys with it and I will show you a quack. He may be an ethical quack, but he is still a quack' (reported in Sherrin[9]).

This view of medicine, although appealing, is not universally accepted. Its most egregious omission is its failure to recognise the ancient, ongoing and contemporary tensions between two traditions of medical practice identified with the mythical characters Asclepius and Hygeia. Asclepius was the son of Apollo, who gained his power through the use of the knife and his understanding of the power of plants to cure illness. The Asclepian tradition sees health as effectively the absence of disease; this tradition recognises that in disease there will be an expectation of disorder and disharmony. The role of the physician is to bring external forces to bear to overcome the disorder and bring the individual back to an ordered state of health.

Hygeia was the daughter of Asclepius (her sister was Panacea). In the Hygeian tradition health is a natural and normal way of things, derived from a state of inner equilibrium and balance.[10] Treatment in this tradition is seen as a way of restoring equilibrium, and the role of the physician is to help to achieve this by re-establishing not only an inner balance between the individual's physical, emotional and spiritual aspects of illness, but also an outer balance between the person and the person's environment.

While it is the Asclepian tradition, with its focus on health as the absence of disease, that is epitomised as the basis of Hippocratic medicine, this denies the diversity of intellectual and social approaches to medicine at that time. Conventional analyses of medicine extract from the Graecian era only those elements that support a rationalist ontological view, assumed by those commentators to be a major asset. Dubos[2] asserts that this tension between the Hygeian and Asclepian traditions has always existed in medicine and continues today. The healthism that characterised the approach to well-being in the US from the 1960s onwards evokes this Hygeian model of health; its emergence can be interpreted as an abreaction away from the Asclepian model espoused then and now by the American Medical Association .

The passing of the Medical Act in 1858, with its establishment of the GMC, can be seen as the crowning glory of the Asclepian tradition for medicine in the UK. The act and the establishment of the GMC professionalised medicine in such a way that doctors, medical doctors, were the only people who could legitimately practice medicine. They were the only people considered to have access to the scientific (and it is assumed value-free) esoteric body of knowledge which was rapidly expanding from that time onwards. The act defined the hierarchy which placed conventional medical practitioners above all others including osteopaths, chiropractors and homeopaths. These were all designated to the second rank known collectively as alternative. Not only this, but the act also defined registration and training for doctors creating a professional class who were to become pivotal in the history and politics of medicine from that time on. Even from within the conventional medical profession defined through this act and the establishment of the GMC subdivisions aligning themselves with these two traditions continued to flourish. It was this act that defined the three branches of medicine, in hierarchical order: hospital specialists, GPs and public health physicians. Hospital doctors had their focus exclusively on disease, which distinguished them from the GPs whose interest remained illness, a broader concept whose important distinctions have best been explored by Kleinman.[11] The public health tradition continued to embrace the Hygeian model with its emphasis on prevention rather than cure, up until recently when their main focus of interest switched to efficiency and effectiveness, both concepts inextricably linked with fiscal constraint.

Ivan Illich[12] continued to fuel this debate with the publication of his powerful *Medical Nemesis* in 1975. Here, he argued that conventional medicine had usurped a monopoly on the interpretation and management of health, well-being, suffering, disability, disease and death, ultimately to the detriment of health itself. Illich defined health broadly as the process of adaptation to growing up, ageing, disease and death, using the coping mechanisms embedded in the culture and traditions of communities.

A second weakness in the conventional history of medicine relates to the assumption that the description of Koch's postulates was in fact value free and morally neutral. Alone among commentators, Greaves[3] has pointed out the flaws in this presentation. Essential to the presentation of Koch's postulates was the understanding that these were a morally free, factual description of real disease entities, which existed out there in the real world. But the relationship between the elements, and in particular between the combination of the clinical and pathological elements as against the causal or germ element, was never equivalent. As early as 1895, Virchow recognised a confusion and circularity in this relationship (see translation by Rather[13]). The only solution to the tension between the elements was to create a hierarchy in which one became dominant; not surprisingly that was the causal (germ) element. From this, the whole interest in germ theory flowed, supported by the rise in laboratory medicine and statistical methods, as well as the central political changes which consolidated the sociological position of scientific medicine as the basis for accepted practice in the UK.

The value-free, morally neutral attributions with which Koch's postulates were imbued transferred themselves to the broader notion of disease, whose positivist conception assumes that diseases are defined solely by real distinct and value-free facts. But even this contention (that diseases are simply factually based and value-free) can be challenged. If diseases were real, value-free and universally describable then one could argue that all societies would agree what constitutes and what does not constitute a disease in the same way that developments in physics are regarded with the same qualities irrespective of the society whose scientists regards them; quarks are the same in London, San Francisco or Delhi.

History is, however, littered with examples of diseases that have come and gone over the years. In the nineteenth century American physicians described a disease which existed only in the population of black slaves, and boasted one central feature, namely that they ran away, it was called drapetonania. This was not the only disease from which slaves could 'suffer', dysaesthesia aethiopica was the name given to a disease found only in slaves with rascal-like behaviour! In World War I the tendency of some soldiers to desert, while conventionally regarded as a criminal offence deserving the death penalty, was described by others as neurasthenia, a weakness of the spirit. Hypotension is regarded as a disease in Germany but not in the UK; spasmophylie is regarded a disease of young adolescent females in France, treatable with repeated intramuscular injections of calcium. In the UK, it is regarded simply as a symptom of anxiety caused by hyperventilation. The American College of Psychiatrists regarded homosexuality as a disease up until 1974, and in contemporary medicine confusion still exists about whether conditions like alcoholism or chronic fatigue syndrome are real disease entities.

The important point about these examples is to underline the argument that a disease is not considered to be a disease simply because the bare facts describing it demand that it be so identified. It is because the society places our value on those facts, and certain societies will place different values on the same facts at different times. As Greaves[3] points out, even broken bones cannot be considered as a universal timeless disease; as recently as the seventeenth century the tradition of binding children's feet in China to make them stay small (a sign of social superiority), often induced fractures, but these were not considered to be pathological, that is a disease, in the conventional understanding of that word.

It is possible then to see the history of medicine as evolving in a way that differs substantially from accepted analyses. It can be seen, we argue, as a continuing tension oscillating between two timeless traditions, the Asclepian and the Hygeian. The evolution of medicine is characterised by diversity in approach, altered radically and unexpectedly by great discoveries, and assisted by fortuitous, but essentially unrelated, developments in disciplines like mathematics and technology. What such a view introduces is the notion that there is no incontrovertible continuous intellectual thread running through the history of medicine; the present position, effectively a hegemony of science in medicine can be challenged. The intention in challenging the conventional view of medical history in this way is not to deconstruct medicine irrevocably, not to encourage an irresponsible disregard for its spectacular if narrow successes. It is simply to open the debate, to encourage re-evaluation and to disabuse those reflecting on such issues of the notion of impregnability in the biomedical concept of clinical practice.

References

1 Porter R (1987) *A Social History of Madness.* Widendfield and Nicolson, London.

2 Dubos R (1960) *The Mirage of Health.* George, Allan and Unwin Limited, London.

3 Greaves D (1996) *Mystery in Western Medicine.* Ashgate Publishing Limited, Aldershot, UK.

4 Phillips ED (1973) *Greek Medicine.* Thames and Hudson, London.

5 Porter R (1997) *The Greatest Benefit to Mankind.* Fontana Press, London.

6 Descartes R (1912) *A Discourse on Method*: m*editations and principles.* J Veitch (trans). Dent and Sons Limited, London.

7 Foucault M (1963) *The Birth of the Clinic.* Tavistock, London.

8 Jewson ND (1976) The disappearance of the sick man from medical causmology, 1770–1870. *Sociology.* **10**: 225–44.

9 Sherrin N (1995) *Oxford Dictionary of Humorous Quotations.* OUP, Oxford.

10 Mitchell A, McCormack M (1998) *The Therapeutic Relationship in Complimentary Health Care.* Churchill, Livingstone, London.

11 Kleinman A (1988) The *Illness Narratives.* Basic Books, New York.

12 Illich I (1975) *Medical Nemesis. The expropriation of health.* Calder and Boyars, London.

13 Rather LJ (1958) *Disease Life and Man.* Stanford University Press, Stanford.

Uniqueness in clinical practice: reflections on suffering

Chapters Two and Three re-evaluated the rise of scientific thinking in medicine, showing how a biomedical approach to clinical practice was consolidated professionally and politically during the nineteenth and the first half of the twentieth centuries. At that time, medical science was seen to work like the other natural sciences and the focus of attention was on specific causality in infectious disease; the prevailing attitude was that all infectious diseases would eventually be controlled completely by preventing the transmission of microbes.

Science and medicine became bound up with each other mainly through technology; the distinction between the two was becoming blurred. The idea of the physician as a scientist emerged, and was generally welcomed. The scientific approach, relying on the new, exciting and, above all, objective technology, was expected to diminish subjectivity and individualism, which were perceived to hinder medical practice. These developments were terribly appealing as they held out the promise of simplicity and clarity; hence the origin of the now mostly discredited attempts at computer-assisted diagnosis developed through the 1960s and 1970s.

But there was an inescapable paradox which emerged simultaneously. Science was dealing with generalities and medicine was dealing with individuals. Science was really solving only half of the problem by providing a invaluable taxonomy for understanding the body and its dysfunction. There was another part to the activity and this involved was dealing with the sick person. This kind of activity, inherently a one-to-one activity, remained inextricably shackled to the individual's skills. Quite simply, subjectivity cannot be banished from the practice of medicine. As the twentieth century progressed, science and technology were trying to simplify sets of circumstances that were inherently complex. Certainty was being manufactured, where doubt continued to confound. Thinking was moving inexorably from objectivity to subjectivity.

Around the middle of the twentieth century, several trends emerged to substantiate this view. First, medicine seemed to have cultural boundaries, even if the natural sciences appeared not to. Secondly, there was a rise in the concept of social responsibility in medicine.

In 1958, a classic paper by Walsh McDermot describing morbidity among the Navajo Indians was published. It served as the first piece of evidence to suggest that medicine may not cross cultural boundaries easily. The paper described how this tribe of Native American Indians suffered from a whole host of complaints – a combination of malnutrition, diarrhoea, respiratory illness – for which no microbial cause could be identified (apart from tuberculosis and otitis media). Dubos,[1] one of the great commentators on these matters, argues that here scientific medicine was meeting its first great obstacle, namely a reluctance on the part of certain populations to accept classical disease theory. Medicine, it seemed, had its cultural boundaries.

Brook *et al.*'s classic paper nearly 30 years later was the first to suggest that cultural differences may affect the way clinicians practice too.[2] They conducted an experiment in which cardio-thoracic surgeons in the US and the UK were exposed to an identical series of clinical vignettes, and asked to evaluate the appropriateness of coronary artery bypass grafting in each case. The surgeons in the US and the UK faced with the same clinical problems adopted quite different intervention strategies (the Americans advocated surgical intervention more frequently). But how to explain this? Were not these doctors all part of the same profession , the same tradition, all positivists at heart? Brook *et al.* were mystified, they ended their article attributing the observed differences in clinical practice to 'cultural differences difficult to quantify'.

A comparison of prescribing in Europe five years later provided further evidence that cultural differences affected the way clinicians' provided medications to their patients. Garrantini and Garratini's *Lancet* paper in 1993[3] described the prescribing habits of doctors in four European countries, Great Britain, France, Germany and Italy. The researchers ranked the 50 most-provided products in these countries into three categories as a function of the scientific evidence for their efficacy. In essence their analysis showed that in the UK, the vast majority of products sold were supported by abundant evidence, while in France and Italy about half the products dispensed lacked any decent research evidence of efficacy. This report assumed, not unreasonably, that for the purposes of prescribing, Europe could be considered as a homogeneous community, as it supported the same biomedical paradigm, shared the same literature and increasingly exchanged its practitioners across its national boundaries.

Throughout the 1950s and 1960s, a second trend emerged to slow the inexorable progress of the notion of the doctor as scientist. This was the rise in the concept of a social responsibility in medicine. The decade between 1950 and 1960 was a very turbulent era for medical schools in the USA. Student activists were demanding that the undergraduate curriculum become more relevant to the poor and the oppressed. Simultaneously, the UK had seen the inception of the NHS, the founding of the Royal College of General Practitioners, which went on to develop a strong sense of social responsibility, and the beginnings of consumer research with the Research Institute for Consumer Affairs report in 1963,[4] shortly before Cartwright and Anderson's[5] seminal work five years later.

So these trends, and the inherent paradox which they illustrated between the generality of science and the individuality of medicine, refocused the view that medicine was as much a moral as it was a technological or scientific pursuit. The view was emerging that the central responsibility of medical professionals in any society was the relief of suffering, a concept that included the role and contribution of science, but went far beyond that. The pendulum of practice had swung too far towards the sciences. It was time to redress the balance.

The emergence of this view, and a strong rational to support it, is well documented in an outstanding book by the American physician and anthropologist Eric Cassell called *The Nature of Suffering and The Goals of Medicine*.[6] Cassell argues here that a technological positivist approach to medical practice, with thinking predicated on Cartesian dualism, actually began to impede the discharge of the ultimate responsibility that any society confers on its medical profession, namely the relief of suffering.

He describes suffering as the state of severe distress associated with events that threaten the intactness of the person, or more precisely what Cassell calls the personhood of the individual. The series of characteristics of personhood defined by Cassell are worth rehearsing here, as they confirm the centrality of individuality, of uniqueness and ultimately of subjectivity in medical practice.

Thus, a person has personality and character. Some people are forgiving, generous and grateful even when faced with severe physical disease, while others will be truculent and disagreeable even in a midst of trivial illnesses. A person has a family and cultural background, in which the beliefs and attitudes that constitute the building blocks of an individual's idea of illness (as a threat to well-being) are formed. The intensity of these connections is exposed by the metaphors often used by folk to describe family members as extensions of the body: 'when my wife died, doctor, it was like losing an arm'. A person has a relationship with himself or herself. Cassell argues that although words like honour and cowardice are rarely used in modern conversation, the concepts still play an important role in describing the individual's attitudes to his or her own conduct when faced with disease. A person has a body *and* a relationship with that body that, in times of good health, can be based on pride in physical or even sexual prowess. But chronic disease can have a devastatingly effect such a perception, so that one comes not to trust one's bowels, one's bladder or one's eyesight. Some women feel that they cannot trust their body at the time of the menstrual period. A person does things, has regular behaviours and defined roles to act out. If a person cannot perform such normal routine activities, that person no longer feels whole. In adult life, roles are sometimes so firmly established that the inability to perform them creates an intense feeling of alienation. Indeed recognition of the alienation experienced by a sick person is regarded by some as a role but makes the work for the primary care doctor unique.[7]

Perhaps most important of all, a person has a perceived future, a series of anticipated expectations that form the basis for hope. MacIntyre, a philosopher with an interest in medicine describes the role of hope thus: hope exists, he says 'precisely in the face of evil which tempts us to despair. The presupposition of hope identifies a belief in a reality that transcends evidence'.[8]

The continuing espousal of scientific rationalism, of the ontological basis of the disease and the presumption of intellectual celibacy in the construction of biomedical knowledge, were the three central characteristics of clinical practice that emerged throughout the twentieth century. Here we argue that this development actually presents a paradox, because it endangers the most fundamental responsibility of practitioners of medicine in any society – the relief of suffering.

The intellectual journey presented in the preceding chapters of this book has re-evaluated objectivity in medicine. In this chapter we present the view that subjectivity cannot be banished from clinical practice. There is a third level of analysis – beyond subjectivity – of clinical practice which examines the role of the self in illness (the patient's self) and the role of the physician as self in practice (the doctor's self); we attach the term interiority to this level. Interiority denotes a deeper layer of understanding of the nature of the interaction between doctor and patient, going beyond objectivity and subjectivity.

Patients do not consult with a doctor just to obtain clinical answers to literal questions. Patients do indeed attend with literal questions for which straightforward biomedical answers will suffice, but they will also attend with metaphorical questions. And when patients attend with physical problems they may also attend with metaphysical problems. In summary, patients come to doctors to make sense of their illness experience.[9] They come for help to incorporate an illness into the narrative structure of their own lives. The narrative as a metaphor for understanding the patient's condition has considerable potential. Doctors have narratives too, this introduces the important idea of reciprocity in the consultation, the idea of mutual influence. There are of course some limitations to the narrative metaphor because of the paradox that life is lived prospectively and a narrative can only be understood retrospectively.

This idea of reciprocity represents the essence of personal significance, a term which denotes the need for a third level of significance beyond the two conventional levels of significance, i.e. statistical (clarifying evidence at the research level) and clinical (clarifying evidence at the population level).[10] Personal significance is defined as the key to the transfer of an idea to, and the evaluation of an idea by, the doctor and the patient together. Personal significance is thus as a dialectic, uniting contributions from the practitioner and the individual patient. The importance of this idea, we argue, lies in its requirement to recognise that the consultation between a sick person and a doctor is a reciprocal activity, in which the contribution of the one will influence the other. Both parties combine different parts of the self in the process. The patient combines the sick self with the normal self (Cassell[6] calls this the intact person); the doctor combines the personal self – combining a unique individual history, along with a history of successes and failures in dealing with illness – with the professional self. The two parties engage each other in a dialogue in which the exchanges are composed of three activities that we describe as integration, evaluation and formulation of response.

Consider first the doctor's role. The initial task for the doctor (vastly under-recognised) takes the form of an interior struggle between the doctor's individual self and the doctor's professional self. The former brings the personal narrative to the task of consulting, the personal history, prejudice, attitudes, fears and aspirations, as well as the weaknesses which we all have as frail human beings. It is, firstly, this individual self which has to integrate with the professional self of the doctor to set the scene for engaging in the consultation.

The second task in a consultation involving the doctor's self is evaluation. Here the task for the doctor is to evaluate both the clinical evidence (from research) and the narrative evidence (obtained by exploring the patient's philosophy of health) and deliver a message that represents a synthesis of these two. The best model for understanding this activity comes from Roger Neighbour's book *The Inner Consultation*.[11] Neighbour argues that doctors carry on an inner consultation when faced with a patient, in which there are two functions. The logical, rational part of the activity is the domain of the Organiser, while the Responder acts in a more intuitive capacity.

We argue that doctors conduct an inner consultation with clinical evidence before forming a response which forms the clinical message. This inner consultation requires the doctor to combine cognitive and evaluative assessments of the evidence. That part of the consultation is of course combined with, and responds to, the evidence that is extracted from the patient's narrative. And the whole activity of evaluation unfolds in a dynamic, continuous and ever-changing relationship with the patient which is reciprocal.

The third task for the doctor, which involves the self, is the formulation of a response. This is where the doctor composes a clinical message to deliver to the patient. A crucial part of this involves the doctor's precise choice of words.

The building blocks of discourse in the most general sense is the metaphor. Metaphors are an integral part of language – even referring to them as building blocks is a metaphor in itself. The precise words which the doctor will choose, the exact metaphors which those words construct, and the meaning thus conveyed to the patient will have a profound effect on the way in which the patient will respond.

The view that a patient attends a consultation as a passive participant, awaiting the transfer of purely medical answers to literal questions, is no longer tenable. A single seminal experiment showing how chronic disease parameters improved in patients who interacted more assertively in their consultations put paid to that doctor-centred idea.[12] The role of the patient, we argue, can be seen as a mirror of the professional's role. Thus, the patient actively participates in the three activities as the basis of the consultation namely, integration, evaluation and formulation. The patient will integrate the cognitive components of the illness experience, that is, what he or she factually knows (either correctly or incorrectly) about the clinical issue, with a personal history or narrative which affects that evaluation. Indeed their decision to present is an outcome of their struggle to reconcile the cognitive and personal narrative aspects of the particular illness experience.

The second activity for the patient's self is the evaluation of the message expressed by the doctor. Here, the self of the patient operates in much the same way as the doctor, again bringing cognitive and evaluative skills to the process. The citizen will attempt to make sense of the factual material, but will simultaneously be evaluating and trying to integrate that message into their life plan. Finally, the patient will formulate a response to the message.

This is possibly the best researched of all the activities that are combined in the consultation. People's attitudes to health are not exclusively logical. An individual's attitude to health and decisions taken about health are determined by how they perceive a particular threat to their health, what they perceive to be the advantages of changing their behaviour in order to accommodate that threat and their perception of how difficult that behavioural change might be.[13]

The beliefs that form attitudes to health are not influenced exclusively by factual material but by personal and family factors and by social and demographic factors. Actions based upon these beliefs are not always rational; they can be emotional or simply habitual.[14] Patients are influenced in the actions that they take by what they think others might expect them to do and by how much importance they attach to that. Kant summed up the position elegantly by saying 'we see things not as they are but rather as we are'.

There is an inescapable interiority in the consultation (i.e. in relation to both participants), and we can benefit from reflecting and researching into what actually goes on inside the minds of both participants. Why do they say what they say? In what way precisely do they say it? These become important questions which address the interaction between the professionals and the patient at the deepest level. This analysis places the relationship between the two players as central to understanding the outcome of the dialogue; it evokes a requirement for connectedness to give meaning to the activity. Connectedness does not simply mean participating in a conversation, it means recognising the meaning of one's own contributions and those of the other, responding to them in a reciprocal way. Seen in this way, the consultation is better seen as a horizontal, not a hierarchical, relationship in which the doctor acts exclusively as a resource.

The analysis also implies that holism in medicine denotes not just the patient but the patient and doctor unit. Doctors can elicit emotional cords for patients, but it works the other way too. It is part of the apprenticeship of doctoring that we learn to protect ourselves from the emotional overdrive of bonding too intensely with scores of ill people. Freud tells us that the tension between empathy and objectivity is in fact paralleled by a tension between empathy and self-protection. Discussions about therapeutic relationships tend to focus on the humanity of the sick person, but doctors and nurses are people too, and this analysis elicits the components of personhood that the professional brings to the consultation.

The central thesis underpinning this analysis is clear, that scientific knowledge and sophisticated technology do not do the work of medical practice. Scientific knowledge constructs instruments that will be employed by human beings, whose guiding principles will be moral as much as technical. Toon,[15] taking this view, argues that moral virtues are prerequisites for proper medical practice. Trustworthiness, self-discipline, humility, tolerance and patience become, in his view, tools which the professional uses as the denominator for any clinical activity. This view, of course, does not exclude science, far from it, the view simply predicates the use of scientific knowledge in the realm of trustworthiness and responsibility. One cannot act responsibly on behalf of a sick person without recourse to science. But the perspective has altered, so that the actions are seen in the light of the practice of human virtues, not just the application of scientific facts.

Trust in others, declares Eric Cassell,[6] is one of the central human solutions to the unbearable uncertainty of being ill. Self-discipline implies a sound degree of self-knowledge with which to discharge one's responsibilities adequately. The information upon which proper action will be based may well include the accurate assessment of technological information, but it will go beyond that to include recognition of what a patient is actually experiencing and the meaning of that experience for them as unique individuals.

This analysis, therefore, places the relationship between the doctor and the patient at the centre of the evaluation of healthcare. But is there any evidence to support this view in the medical literature? In Chapter Five, we review the evidence that supports the view that there is a therapeutic component to this kind of relationship, with discernible health gains for the patient when it is present, and identifiable risks in its absence.

References

1 Dubos R (1960) *The Mirage of Health*. George Allen and Unwin Limited, London.

2 Brook RH, Park RE, Winslow CM *et al.* (1988) Diagnosis and treatment of coronary disease: a comparison of doctors' attitudes in the USA and the UK. *Lancet*. **189**: 7550–3.

3 Garratini S, Garratini L (1993) Pharmaceutical prescribing in four European countries. *Lancet*. **342**: 1191–2.

4 Research Institute for Comsumer Affairs (1963) *General Practice: a consumer commentary*. A report prepared for the Consumer Policy Service. Policies Studies Institute, London.

5 Cartwright A, Anderson R (1968) *Patients and Their Doctors : a study of general practice*. Routledge and Kegan Paul, London.

6 Cassell E (1991) *The Nature of Suffering and the Goals of Medicine*. OUP, Oxford.

7 Broodie H (1991) What does the primary care physician do that makers a difference? In: M Stewart (ed.) *Primary Care Research: traditional and innovative approaches*. Sage Publications, Newbury Park, CA.

8 MacIntyre A (1979) Seven traits for designing our descendants. *The Hastings Centre Report*. **9**: 5–7.

9 Heath I (1995) *The Mystery of General Practice*. Nuffield Hospitals Provincial Trust, London.

10 Sweeney KG, MacAulay, D, Pereira Gray DJ (1998) Personal significance: the third dimension. *Lancet*. **351**: 134–6.

11 Neighbour R (1987) *The Inner Consultation*. MTP Press Ltd, Lancaster, UK.

12 Kaplan SH, Greenfield S, Ware JE (1989) Assessing the effect of physician patient interaction on the outcomes of chronic disease. *Med Care*. **27** (Suppl.): S125.

13 Fishbein M *et al.* (1975) *Belief, Attitude Intention and Behaviour*. Wiley, New York.

14 Becker MH (1974) The health belief model and the sick role behaviour. *Health Education Monographs.* **2**: 409–19.

15 Toon P (1999) *Towards a Philosophy of General Practice: a study of the virtuous practitioner, Occasional Paper 78.* Royal College of General Practitioners, London.

CHAPTER FIVE

Doctors and patients: the therapeutic relationship

So far we have developed two propositions. First, we argued in favour of a re-evaluation of the role of science in medicine by describing a legitimate inquiry into the philosophical and historical bases of clinical practice. Secondly, we analysed the consultation between a patient and a doctor in a way that displayed its complex evolutionary and elusive nature. We advocated a deeper reflection of the interior experience of both participants in this reciprocal activity. This analysis should have a clear purpose. Where, then, is this leading? Quite simply, the purpose of this inquiry is to explore better ways of consulting, which will benefit patients. But is it a realistic possibility that the relationship developed between a doctor and a patient in a series of consultations could produce a real benefit, i.e. a determinable health gain, for the patient? In this chapter we look at the evidence that supports this possibility, namely of a therapeutic outcome to the relationship between the doctor and the patient.

In the last 150 years research in medicine has focused mainly on biomedical science, reflecting an implicit acceptance of scientific positivism. Interest in the non-biological aspects of clinical practice has had no sustained history but rather is characterised by peaks and troughs of attention. But the debate is not by any means new; for centuries, medical writers and thinkers have debated the importance of relationships in medicine, of good communication and of trust as the basis of the clinical interaction. Porter[1] attributes the earliest descriptions of the values which derive from fostering good relationships with patients to Hippocrates. 'Make frequent visits' declared Hippocrates 'and enquire into all particulars. Cultivate prognosis, so that men will have confidence to entrust themselves to such a physician' (pp. 59–61).[1] His contemporaries Plato and Rufus of Ephesus also make passing reference to the importance of good communication in fostering the doctor–patient relationship.[2]

Although during the Renaissance there was no clearly sustained interest in the mechanics of the doctor–patient relationship, the whole basis of clinical interaction rested upon the careful communication in the history taking (probably faute de mieux, the physicians had little else to make use of). Spirituality, however, was seen as integral to the human condition, both in health and disease. 'The human body was created for the sake of the soul', wrote the Venetian surgeon Alessandro Benedetti (1450–1512), 'and stands erect among other animals as established by divine nature and reason so that it might look up more comfortably (Porter, p. 169[1]). And, when two centuries ago Descartes (1596–1650) recounted his most famous dictum, 'Cogito ergo sum', he was later to be countered by Jean Jacques Rousseau (1712–1778), who advocated the quintessentially Romantic view: I 'thought before I felt'.[3]

Later still, in literature and poetry, the Romantics continued to develop a strong tradition countering the Cartesian dualism, which dominated medical thought throughout the seventeenth and eighteenth centuries. Wordsworth advocated a holistic view when referring in the *Tables Turned* to, 'our meddling intellect mishaps the beauteous form of things, we murder to dissect'.[4] One hundred and fifty years later TS Elliott contributed to this centuries-old debate with a plea for reconciliation and dialectic unification 'where is the life we have lost in living? Where is the wisdom we have lost in knowledge? Where is the knowledge we have lost in information?'[5] At least in poetry, writers continued to explore the historical tensions between the Asclepian and Hygeian traditions of medicine referred to earlier.

Closer to clinical medical practice, Freud was the first to introduce a vocabulary that hinted at potentially therapeutic, as well as disastrous, consequences of the interaction between a therapist and a patient. His definitions of transference, the development of an emotional attitude towards analysis on the part of the client, and counter-transference (its reciprocal) represented an important formalisation of the thinking about these relationships for the first time.

But it is in the second half of the twentieth century that a continuing tradition of enquiry into the potential benefit in the doctor–patient relationship really began to develop. In the 1950s pioneering work by the psychotherapist Michael Balint (1957) first began to capture the processes that underpinned and explained the interaction between *The Doctor, His Patient and The Illness* – the title of his seminal text. What Balint drew attention to most of all was the skill of listening, which he considered to be of paramount importance in the consultation. For Balint listening meant not just tuning in to what the patient was saying, or indeed was implying in an unspoken way, but also developing a greater awareness of the doctor's self . Balint puts it this way, 'Listening requires a new skill necessitating a considerable though limited change in personality. While discovering in himself an ability to listen to things in his patient that are barely spoken because the patient himself is barely aware of them, the doctor soon starts listening to the same kind of language in himself'.[6] Balint was the first to confront and utilise the doctor's emotional reaction to the patient; he advocated recognising the phenomenon of counter-transference and using it to the patient's advantage. In turn, this should allow the doctor to develop, as the process increased self-awareness. Using his background as an analytical psychologist, Balint helped the doctors who participated in his now famous seminars to recognise the importance of unconscious motivation in human behaviour. Doctors are people too, they come to consultations with their own baggage, the emotions, beliefs and experiences that make them who and what they are. What doctors as a profession had failed to realise was the extent to which this personal baggage could influence their professional behaviour. Increased self-awareness allowed the doctor to develop what Balint described as the 'apostolic function', that is a function going beyond the conventional task-oriented biomedical role to create a therapeutic milieu in which the patient could be helped.

Here Balint was acknowledging the influence that patients' suffering could have on the physician as a person, the inescapable fact that the majority of the patients they were seeing had incurable illnesses, with which their interventionist style of medical education was ill-equipped to deal. Their gradually increasing distress, the inexorable dilemmas in which many of them lived out their lives, influenced by unalterable social conditions or disastrous, but inescapable, personal relationships, produced a response in the physician. Either one could fail to recognise this, in which case one usually distanced oneself from this aspect of the problem, focusing exclusively on the 'safe' scientific parts, or one could confront it and make use of it in good clinical practice, which we know is influenced by emotions and relationships. We argue that here Balint was advocating that the doctor adopted and developed a healer role 'walking with the patient' as Jean Vanier the founder of L'Arche, a network of communities for the intellectually disabled, puts it.[7] This phrase implies a lack of judgement, coupled with and reinforced by a commitment to the relationship with the patient and an ability to offer impartial therapeutic insight into it.

A decade after the publication of Balint's book, the first experimental evidence that relationships could have an effect on an individual's health began to appear in peer-reviewed journals. In 1967, the *BMJ* published a paper by a Welsh GP, Dewi Rees and his research assistant, Sylvia Lutkins, formally entitled The Mortality of Bereavement, but now universally referred to as 'Dying of a Broken Heart'.[8] The study explored the effect of bereavement on close relatives. The researchers compared the mortality at one year in a group of close relatives of a deceased person with a control group living in the same area who had not suffered bereavement. Their principal finding surprised a sceptical and conservative medical audience. The researchers noted a seven-fold increase in risk of death the bereaved group. Rees and Lutkins summarised their findings poetically: 'He first deceased, she for a little tried; To live without him; liked it not and died' (Sir Henry Wotton).

Although the medical literature is relatively weak in this area, health psychologists have developed a stronger literature which constitutes a body of evidence supporting the view that physical health can be linked to the quality of interpersonal relationships. And although this literature does not cover precisely the doctor–patient relationship, it does merit some consideration here.

First of all there is a large number of studies that link health benefit to the actual existence of relationships, of which that described by Berkman[9] serves as one example. A series of studies has examined the health benefits deriving from stable marriages. In loving marriages, husbands reported less angina, as they also did in the same study, when family conflict was the variable, the less the intrafamily conflict, the less the husbands reported angina.[10] But interpreting these studies can be tricky; here, it could have been the case that husbands who experienced less loving marriages and more conflict (and also experienced more angina) may have had only themselves to blame, for example by being hostile – and that it was this that caused their angina. A curious set of studies looked at newly married couples, and was able to extract data from blood samples that were analysed for immune competence and physiological markers of stress. In a series of 90 newly wed couples, the exhibition of hostile or negative behaviours was associated with serial decrements in immune status as well as elevation of blood pressure, ACTH, growth hormone and adrenaline.[11]

The nature of parent–child relationships seem to be associated with health status in adult life too. Thomas *et al.*'s study[12] established that medical students who reported experiencing less warm relationships with their own parents when young had a higher chance of developing cancer 25 years later. Simply having a relationship which a participant can describe as intimate appears to be associated with better overall mental and physical health.[13] This is probably the key message to extract from this body of literature; the very fact that we interact with others, and to some extent the way in which those interactions play out, affects our health. And although this evidence should not be extrapolated directly to health, there are sufficient similarities between the context in which these relationship studies occur, and the context in which patients and their doctors develop their interpersonal relationships to at least encourage healthcare researchers to continue to study the nature of the doctor–patient relationship.

From the 1970s onwards, evidence continued to emerge in the mainstream medical literature of the interaction of the body and the mind in health in a way that really demanded a change from the prevailing medical metaphor of the body as machine to a new metaphor, that of the embodied mind.[14] Depression occurring in a particularly severe form after childbirth was recognised, as well as a milder form following viral illnesses. In 1989, a study in the USA gave the first evidence of a proxy measure of benefit when patients were coached to interact better with their physician, and thus develop a better 'therapeutic' relationship.[15] In their study, Kaplan and his team identified a group of patients with common chronic diseases, such as diabetes and high blood pressure, assessed how well-controlled their diseases were, and discussed with the patients how they got on with their physicians. They coached the patients to interact more positively with their doctors, demonstrating techniques of assertive participation in the consultations.

As a consequence of their coaching, the team noted much better control of blood pressure in the hypertensives, and less variation in the blood sugars of the diabetic patients. For their part, the doctors did not seem to like it much; when the team tried to obtain funding for a bigger study to confirm their findings, they were unsuccessful.

In the 1990s, links between unhappiness in childhood and poor health in adulthood began to emerge, for example linking slower rates of growth in children who had experienced a traumatic childhood.[16] The consequences of adverse life events in childhood appear to linger and influence health well into adulthood. Brunner *et al.*[17] reported a study on possible determinants of plasma fibrinogen, a key contributing factor in the development of heart disease. The researchers knew that higher plasma fibrinogen levels were found in people from lower socioeconomic groups, and although smoking certainly contributed to this gradient, it could not by itself explain the extent of the difference. As part of an earlier study the same researchers had found a curious link between the risk of heart disease and the perception of having little control at work. The group carried out a cross-sectional survey of over 2000 civil servants, measuring their plasma fibrinogen, and obtaining information about their childhood (educational achievements and parents occupation) and the extent to which they could control their work environment (assessed by personnel managers). They formed two conclusions: first, measures of childhood environment, namely educational status and adult height (as a measure of overall physical well-being) were inversely linked to plasma fibrinogen;

secondly, monotony, low control and under-utilisation of skills at work was similarly related to higher levels of this cardiac risk factor. Fibrinogen, the team argued, could be the marker for the biological pathways mediating the inverse social economic gradient in coronary disease.

Experiencing adverse life events seems to be linked with breast cancer too. Several studies have showed that women who had experienced life stress were at greater risk of developing the disease. In one study, all severe life events, and coping with the stress of adverse events by confronting them, increased the possibility of developing cancer of the breast by a factor of three.[18] And for those suffering breast cancer, evidence from a randomised control trial showed that emotional support from a nurse significantly reduced morbidity in women undergoing breast care surgery.[19] Weiss and Sunder[20] suggested that the link between adverse life events and the onset of serious illness could be attributed to alterations in the immune status; their review clearly showed that stress acts as an inhibitor of the immune response, particularly diminishing natural killer cell activity.

Taken together, this evidence from the general medical literature begins to support the view that the interaction between two people can itself act as a benefit or indeed disbenefit with important implications for health, including an increase in the risk of life-threatening diseases. As far as general practice is concerned hard evidence of the benefit from a doctor–patient relationship is more difficult to come by. However, proxy measures can be found in the literature on continuity of care from a personal GP. For decades continuity of care has been perceived as a desirable attribute of general practice, it has been included in all the main definitions of general practice, such as the Royal College of General Practitioners or the Leeuwenhorst Working Party. Both doctors and patients seem to like it.[21,22] Continuity of care improves both patient satisfaction with a general practice service, but also more importantly improves their compliance with medical advice. It seems that patients who get to know their GP (and by implication are able to develop a good relationship with the doctor) are more likely to take their pills as advised.[23] The benefits seem to work both ways; an improved knowledge of the patient's lifestyle correctly interpreted can help doctors to asses how an illness is developing and how serious it might be.[24]

The opposite also appears to hold true. In a study of patients who did not receive continuity of care, the very lack of continuity of care was associated with additional morbidity, an increase in the number of relationship problems which the patient discussed, an increase in the number of difficult consultations with the doctor and, finally, an increase in the number of appointments which these patients attended, or indeed made and failed to attend. This group who failed to received continuity of care used open access clinics more, particularly accident and emergency, which increased the cost of providing healthcare to them.[25] And when patients change their doctors, it is often because of a perceived breakdown in the relationship. When they take things further by suing their doctors the rationale is not simply to obtain redress for an injury, but rather to acknowledge insensitive handling, poor communication and an overall breakdown in relationships.[26] If having a good relationship with your doctor seems to improve your health, having a bad one at least raises the suspicion of poorer health.

The case is by no means watertight, but there is enough evidence in the medical literature to suggest the strong possibility that patients can derive a health gain from developing good personal relationships with a doctor. For GPs, the importance of this cannot be under-estimated, as their overall responsibility embraces, but goes well beyond, the mere application of biomedical evidence. Iona Heath[27] has identified three key roles for the GP, interpreting a patient's story, guarding against over-medicalisation and witnessing suffering. This evokes the important distinction between a disease and an illness; the former is a narrower biomedical reconfiguration of a patient's story, which necessarily abstracts certain, but not all key, elements of the experience and attaches a significance and an importance to them, the nature of which might well elude the sick person (who may not actually agree with the interpretation anyway).[28] And one can argue that in general practice, doctors rely less on biomedical science either as a diagnostic aid or as a means of intervening than in any other branch of medicine. KB Thomas,[29] in his MD to the University of Liverpool estimated that 50% of what a GP sees cannot be classified in a recognised biomedical taxonomy, and possibly as much 75% cannot be cured, in the literal sense of that word. Does this imply that general practice is different? Should GPs rely on their ability to develop relationships more, since they cannot rely on 'objective' biomedical knowledge as much as their specialist colleagues? Professor Ian McWhinney[30] of the Centre for Family Practice at the University of Ontario certainly argues this, and went as far as to entitle his eponymous lecture to the Annual General Meeting of the Royal College of General Practitioners in 1988 'The importance of being different'. He described four differences. General practice, McWhinney argued, is the only discipline that defines itself in terms of relationships. As a result, GPs tend to think in terms of individual patients, not generalised disease categories; and as a consequence of this, they are forced to transcend the restrictive dualistic division of mind and body, which has so dominated conventional medical thinking for the last two centuries, and embrace another metaphor for the body. The embodied mind becomes the central theme and thinking has to develop organismically, accepting uncertainty and an inherent instability in biological systems. Crucially, thinking and feeling come to be seen as reciprocal activities.

The scene is thus set to explore the next two sections of this book. In Part Two we explore the idea of the physician healer, that is the idea that the interaction which a doctor conducts with a patient can be inherently therapeutic. Conventionally, such effects have been collated under the term placebo – a term much maligned or at best ignored by mainstream medicine, but which we will argue can confer substantial benefits for both the patient and the doctor. In Part Three we explore how the doctor can best recognise and develop generic skills as a physician healer.

References

1   Porter R (1998) *The Greatest Benefit to Mankind*. Fontana Press, London.

2   Irwin WG, Mclelland R, Love AHG (1989) Communications skills

training for medical students: an integrated approach. *Med Educ.* **23**: 367–94.

3   Encarta (1996) Section on romanticism. Microsoft Electronic Encyclopedia, USA. Microsoft copyright.

4   Wordsworth W (1947) Tables turned. In: *The Poems of Wordsworth*. Macmillan Press, London.

5   Elliott TS (1934) The rock. In: *Collected Poems, 1909–1962*. Faber and Faber, London.

6   Balint M (1957) *The Doctor, His Patient and The Illness*. Pitman Paperbacks, London.

7   Vanier J (1998) *Becoming Human*. Anansi, Toronto.

8   Reese WD, Lutkins SG (1967) The mortality of bereavement. *BMJ.* **4**: 13–16.

9   Berkman L F (1995) The role of social relations in health promotion. *Psychosom Med.* **57**: 245–54.

10   Medalie JH, Goldbourt U (1976) Unrecognised myocardial infarction: 5 year incidence mortality and risk factors. *Ann Intern Med.* **84**: 523–31.

11   Kiecolt-Glaser JK, Marlakey WB, Chee M *et al.* (1993) Negative behaviour during marital conflicts associated with immunological down regulation. *Psychosom Med.* **55**: 395–409.

12   Thomas CB, Duszynski KR, Shaffer JW (1979) Family attitudes reported in youth as potential predictors of cancer. *Psychosom Med.* **41**: 287–302.

13   Reis HT (1984) Social interaction and well being. In: Duck SW (ed.) *Personal Relationships: repairing personal relationships*, Vol 5. Academic Press, London.

14   Varela FI, Thompson E, Rosch E (1993) *The Embodied Mind: cognitive science and human experience.* MIT Press, Cambridge, MA.

15   Kaplan SH, Greenfield S, Ware JE (1989) Assesing the effects of patient-physician interaction on the outcomes of chronic diseases. *Med Care.* **27**: 110–27.

16   Montgomery SM, Bartley MJ, Wilkinson RG (1997) Family conflict and slow growth. *Arch Dis Childhood.* **4**: 326–30.

17   Brunner E, Davey Smith G, Marmot M *et al.* (1996) Childhood social circumstances and psychosocial and behavioural factors as determinants of plasma fibrinogen. *Lancet.* **347**: 1008–13.

18 Chen C, David A, Nunnerley H *et al.* (1995) Adverse life events and breast cancer: case control study. *BMJ.* **311**: 1527–30.

19 McArdle J, David GW, McArdle CS *et al.* (1996) Psychological support for patients undergoing breast cancer surgery: a randomised study. *BMJ.* **312**: 813–17.

20 Weiss JM, Sunder S (1992) Effects of stress on cellular immune responses in animals. *Rev Psychiat.* **11**: 145–80.

21 Roland M, Mayor V, Morris R (1986) Factors associated with achieving continuity of care in general practice. *J R Coll Gen Practitioners.* **36**: 102–4.

22 Freeman GK, Richards SC (1993) Is personal continuity of care compatible with free choice of doctor? *Br J Gen Pract.* **43**: 493–7.

23 Attlinger P, Freeman G (1981) General practice compliance study: is it worth being a personal doctor? *BMJ.* **282**: 1192–4.

24 Wright A (1988). *Depression: recognition and management in general practice.* Royal College of General Practitioners, London.

25 Sweeney K, Pereira Gray DJ (1995) Patients who do not receive continuity of care from their general practitioner. *Br J Gen Pract.* **45**: 153–8.

26 Vincent C, Young M, Phillips A (1994) Why do people sue doctors? A study of patients and relatives taking legal action. *Lancet.* **343**: 1609–13.

27 Heath I (1995) T*he Mystery of General Practice.* Nuffield Hospitals Provincial Trust, London.

28 Kleinman A (1988) *The Illness Narratives.* Basic Books, New York.

29 Thomas KB (1974) The temporary dependant patient. *BMJ.* **I**: 59–65.

30 McWhinney I (1988) The importance of being different. *Br J Gen Pract.* 46: 433–6.

PART TWO

Placebo theory and research: the physician healer

Michael Dixon

CHAPTER SIX

Using the placebo effect

The self-healing process is seen most clearly when patients get better having taken a remedy that is known to be ineffective – a *placebo*. Such healing effects do not need to be mediated by an inert substance/placebo but can occur as a direct effect of the doctor/patient interaction – as a *placebo effect*. The physician healer should aim to maximise his/her use of the placebo effect as this will maximise the patient's ability to heal him/herself. Research on placebos and the placebo effect therefore provides a lot of useful evidence as to how we can become better physician healers.

Many doctors will have an initial antipathy towards the concept of 'exploiting the placebo effect' very much like the modern antipathy towards prescribing placebos. The argument would be that we are there to provide active treatments and procedures, which distinguishes modern medicine from charlatanism. Much of the problem lies in the word 'placebo', which should probably be re-termed 'the self-healing or human effect'.

One of the authors (MD) presented a paper at the Fifth Complementary Health Symposium[1] in Exeter in December 1998, which was a report of some scientifically controlled research into the effectiveness of spiritual healers. The results seemed impressive. The patients in both study and control groups had been chronically ill with a number of diseases for an average of five years and had not been helped by any previous conventional or complementary treatments. The results showed that 80% of study patients showed improvement, with 50% showing significant improvement, whereas control patients showed no improvement. The study group also showed a significant improvement in general well-being (anxiety and depression scores). The research did not attempt to dissect out whether spiritual healers were helping through a 'placebo' effect or whether (as they believed) the effect was due to specific transfer of energy at the time of healing. To physician healers, anyway, the debate is irrelevant as the main finding in the study was that one person (without medical training) could catalyse a significant healing response in 50% of patients who had been ill for some time without using anything other than her presence. Placebo or miracle? Does it matter as long as the patients get better? The second paper of that same symposium suggested that the effects of spiritual healing were largely due to a placebo, having found that patients separated from the healer by a screen showed no greater improvement than patients who believed that the healer was the other side of the screen when he/she was not.[2] If both pieces of research are true and if healers can exert a 50% improvement rate in patients, which is purely placebo, then how much more of an effect should an experienced doctor be able to exert? Maximising the placebo effect is not a question of deceiving nor is it an artificial effect. Indeed catalysing a self-healing process in a patient through real self-engendered physiological changes can be a much more robust treatment than trying to effect the patient's recovery using external drugs and procedures. It is also a far more 'natural' treatment and this is conceptually important for many of our patients. Placebo research is thus very pertinent to the question of how we can improve our ability to heal our patients.

What conditions respond to placebos?

Over 40 years ago, Beecher[3] found that there was an average placebo response of 35.2% in a review covering 15 placebo studies and 1082 patients. Since then marked placebo effects have been found in a large range of conditions including angina, congestive cardiac failure, hypertension, peptic ulcer disease, rheumatoid arthritis, osteoarthritis, pain, hay fever, headaches, cough, multiple sclerosis, anxiety, depression, phobias and dementia.

We know that placebos can have a marked effect on the cardiovascular system. In 1933 a study of patients who had had *angina* for two years showed that 38% of patients given an 'inert' substance showed improvement in their symptoms. Indeed the 'inert' substance provided the same improvement as the other 15 'active' drugs that were tested, yet the conclusion at the time was that the patients treated with inactive substance had been party to some miraculous and spontaneous remission of the symptoms.[4] It has since become clear that angina is very responsive to placebo. A more recent study in 1988 showed no significant difference between treatment for angina by a drug that is generally regarded as effective (Iso-Mack-Retard 20) and placebo.[5] Significant differences between the two groups, totalling 45 patients, were only obtained by excluding 15 placebo-sensitive patients. Placebo operations tend to be even more effective than placebo drugs. For instance, a now redundant operation for angina (internal mammary artery ligation) was reported as providing at least 60% relief for pain in its time, but was discontinued when a 'placebo' operation, which simply involved cutting the skin showed a similar 60% success rate.[6]

Congestive *cardiac failure* has also been shown to respond to placebo treatment. A study in 1992 reviewed 24 patients with moderately severe congestive cardiac failure, and compared those taking a placebo with those not taking one.[7] The placebo group showed an 81-second improvement in exercise duration and a statistically significant improvement in functional class by 27% above baseline, which was not shown for the non-placebo group. A placebo effect on *blood pressure* was shown in a study in the *BMJ* in 1988 on the effectiveness of paranormal healing.[8] Fifteen weeks of treatment on placebo showed a mean reduction in blood pressure of 17.1 (systolic) and 8.3 (diastolic). Another study looked at the effect on 90 hypertensive patients of a placebo tablet given daily for 8 days.[9] Thirty per cent of patients showed a significant decrease in blood pressure by around 10% (as opposed to 20% showing a significant increase of around 8%) and 25% showed a significant reduction in heart rate. A study in 1992 showed that hypertensive patients can be conditioned to respond to placebo.[10] An 'atenolol placebo' given after active atenolol produced a significantly greater anti-hypertensive response and slower heart rate than if all treatment was ceased.

Peptic ulcers, which have enormous cost implications following the introduction of histamine antagonists and proton-pump inhibitors, have also been shown to be responsive to placebo treatment. A multicentre trial involving 172 patients with benign gastric ulcer showed a 45% response to placebo, which was confirmed by endoscopy at 6 weeks.[11] Patients on active treatment (Cimetidine) showed 65% response at 6 weeks. The implication is not that we should stop using these powerful drugs on all patients but that we should try to find out the characteristics of the 45% of patients, who do not seem to need them.

A strong placebo response has also been recorded for tinnitus, showing a 40% improvement.[12] Patients with *Ménière's disease* treated with an endolymphatic sac mastoid shunt or with the placebo operation (mastoidectomy), both showed a 70% improvement in terms of hearing according to both patients' and investigators' evaluations, which continued for at least 3 years.[13] The investigators concluded that the improvement was 'most likely caused by a placebo effect'.

There is also a strong placebo effect in *migraine* and a review of several studies has shown 62% of 188 subjects improving by 75% after 4 weeks on placebo with a continued effect after this.[14]

A placebo effect in *multiple sclerosis* (MS) has also been shown in a trial which compared recombinant alpha 2 interferon with placebo in a double-blind trial.[15] Interferon is known to increase natural killer cell activity and both interferon and placebo increased natural killer cell activity during the first week of treatment. Both short-term and long-term clinical improvement (at one year) was noted in the placebo group. Interestingly, a similar incidence of adverse reactions to treatment was reported by both groups. This is a common finding in placebo research and bears out the hypothesis that treatments without any side-effects at all are suspect! The ability of placebo in this study to increase natural killer cell activity may have implications beyond MS as such cells may represent a first line of defence against malignant cells. Indeed, a study in the *Lancet* in 1989 looked at 86 women with metastatic *carcinoma of the breast*, who were randomly allocated to a control group or a treatment group which received group therapy and which looked at coping mechanisms in cancer and self-hypnosis for pain.[16] The treatment group survived longer (mean 36.6 months) than the control group (10.8 month) and the result was statistically significant ($p < 0.0001$). Another study on patients with Hodgkin's or non-Hodgkin's lymphoma showed increased survival at five years for those who had had relaxation training and hypnotherapy for the control of chemotherapy-induced nausea and sickness.[17] Such psychological intervention would be considered as a 'placebo' in orthodox medical research on cancer and thus even cancer may be amenable to the 'placebo effect'.

Psychological problems also respond well to placebo. For instance, there is a 67% placebo response for *dementia*.[18] A substantial placebo response has also been shown repeatedly in depression. The classic Medical Research Council (MRC) trial on *depression* involving carefully diagnosed depressives showed a 39% response at 4 weeks and a 20% response at 6 months.[19] Another large-scale clinical trial covering 555 patients by the USA National Institute for Mental Health concluded that active drugs made very little difference to the outcome of patients with depression (only 10% of the variance).[20] In this trial females aged under 40 years and 'hostile depressives' did particularly well on placebo. More recent studies on depression have shown that the placebo effect is more marked in acute, rather than chronic depression and where there has been a good previous response to antidepressant treatment.[21] As we shall see both these findings fit well with the conditioning theory of the placebo effect. A visit to Lourdes, which many doctors would consider to be no more than a placebo, was shown to decrease anxiety and depression at a statistically significant level when measured one month and ten months after the pilgrims had returned.[22]

A double-blind trial on 41 patients with *panic disorders* showed a 34% response to placebo, defined as a reduction in the number of panic attacks to zero. Patients responding to placebo appeared to have less other psychopathology and to be less help-seeking than those who did not respond.[23] A single-blind placebo trial of 44 agoraphobic patients over a two-week period showed a statistically significant (but not clinically significant) reduction in panic and phobic symptoms.[24] By the end of ten weeks, however, 20–30% of the patients could be classified as marked responders on key panic and phobic measures. The results showed that panic, anxiety and depression were helped early by placebo, but it required time for the phobic symptoms to improve significantly.

Even *schizophrenia*, it seems, responds to placebo. Haemodialysis was once thought to be a useful therapy when initial studies showed that 23% of 49 patients responded. When the effects of actual and placebo dialysis were compared with a further 114 patients in a double-blind experiment, it was found that the marked improvement in 21% of the patients did not differ significantly between those schizophrenics receiving placebo and those receiving actual haemodialysis.[25] It was concluded that the patients had 'favourably reacted to the strong healing involvement'. This high placebo response clearly has major implications for when we should intervene with some of the new expensive pharmaceutical interventions that are available.

Conversely, there seems to be almost no placebo effect, when placebo is given to patients with *obsessive-compulsive disorder*.[26] This might infer that rigidity of mind makes a patient immune to the placebo effect and that if you wished to unlock the placebo effect you may need to create a safe environment, where the rigid thinker can surmount his or her self-imposed boundaries. The risk here, of course, is that the rigid thinker will approach the new paradigm, whether it be eastern philosophy or psychological theory, with the same attention to detail that will once again shut out the voice within!

There has also been a lot of research showing a marked and complex placebo effect in pain relief. For instance a double-blind trial on patients with pain from bony metastases showed that placebo was effective for 57% of patients with a mean improvement of 30–40%. The improvement was maintained after the seven-day treatment and it was found that responders tended to be younger than non-responders.[27] A study on pain following dental surgery compared ultrasound therapy, mock ultrasound therapy and self-massage. Self-massage (e.g. no treatment group) showed no improvement, but placebo ultrasound showed a beneficial analgesic and anti-inflammatory effect – equal to that of real ultrasound. In particular facial swelling, trismus, pain and C-reactive protein were all reduced significantly.[28] In a similar study, placebo TENS was given following appendicectomy was shown to be as effective as active TENS. The placebo provided a significant decrease in both pain severity and analgesic intake. It is interesting to note that having proved that placebo TENS was effective, this paper in the *Annals of the Royal College of Surgeons* concluded that 'its use in this situation cannot be recommended'. In the name of ethical and intellectual honesty, we feel obliged to offer our patients treatments, which may sometimes be more expensive and harmful than placebos that work as well.

It has been estimated that placebo can provide the pharmacological effect of diamorphine 5 mg in treating the pain of tooth extraction.[29] It also seems that placebo is around 55% as efficient as active analgesia, whatever the analgesic.[30] This strange finding has been reported in a review of 17 double-blind studies on aspirin, codeine and morphine where placebo efficiency varied only between 54 and 56%.

It is clear from all these studies that placebo has wide-ranging effects in medicine in a wide range of conditions and must be affecting not only symptoms, but also physiological processes. What do we know about the various factors that contribute to the effectiveness of the placebo effect?

Factors which determine the effectiveness of the placebo effect

Which patients?

Attempts to predict which patients are going to respond to placebo have been largely unsuccessful. There seems to be a core of 11–13% of patients, who will almost always respond to placebo medications.[30] They have been described as 'having good social judgement, being outgoing and enthusiastic, verbally and socially skilled with vague thinking tendencies or introverted, less socially dominant, more passive with lower self-confidence and having lower self-sufficiency, high anxiety and increased religiosity'.[31] Age seems to be a factor in the placebo response with two studies[20,26] showing that younger people respond better than the older generation and are more compliant with medication.[32]

Balint[33] predicted that neurotics and those with an increased level of psychopathology would respond less well to placebo and recent research[23] certainly agrees with this view. In angina, for instance, it has been shown that the placebo effect is inversely related to neuroticism as measured on the Eysenck Personality Inventory.[14] Although double-blind studies have confirmed that neurotics respond poorly to placebos (when they are unaware that they are placebos), another study[34] showed, rather bizarrely that their neurotic symptoms were helped by sugar pills in 14 out of 15 patients when they knew that this was all that they were getting! Neurotics may be looking for the sort of control that is offered by taking a medication that they know to be inert – this allows them to put their own house in order and keep control. Alternatively, they may simply require the sort of self-approbation that is implied when a doctor gives a patient an explicit placebo. Few people would argue that it is ethically wrong to give a placebo when you have actually told the patient that it is a placebo. Nevertheless, the effectiveness of sugar pills, when known to be so, should alert us strongly to the probability that, when patients want to heal themselves, they can be helped to do so by the simplest of cues.

As doctors, we are often tempted to give placebo to our most neurotic and demanding patients. This may be why we generally underestimate the placebo effect, which will be stronger in those with organic rather than functional disease and in those who are 'normal' rather than neurotic. Yet 'normal' patients with functional disease are the very patients that most doctors would feel it important to give effective, clinically proven medicines – where the placebo effect is likely to go unnoticed.

The attitude and motivation of the patient are predictably important, and both field and laboratory studies have shown the importance of motivation in influencing the perception of symptom change.[35] In a trial of 44 patients in which 50% showed significant improvement in their mental illness, the researchers concluded that 'favourable patient attitude towards the use of chemotherapy held a strong relationship to outcome'.[36] Strangely perhaps, hostility seems to be a factor in improving the placebo response.[20] Studies on compliance, which show that nearly half our patients do not take them as pre-scribed, have shown that motivation to recover and the patient's attitude towards their illness are important influences on the level of compliance.[31]

The message to the GP is clear. He/she must concentrate on the attitude and motivation of the patient – any improvements are likely to make the treatment more effective. Indeed our potential to alter the patient's perception of his/her disease may indirectly have far more beneficial consequences than any more direct therapeutic attempts to alter the course of disease.

There is an increasing concentration in modern general practice on information but information, can do nothing it if does not affect the attitude, motivation and emotions of the patient. All of us have witnessed, first hand, the effects of an inspirational teacher but their effects were not created by black and white information but by the energy, enthusiasm and wisdom, which they used to produce their message. It is not the message the therapist gives that matters but that which the patient receives.

What sort of doctors?

Predictably, the attitude and motivation of the doctor are important. This is why the first to receive a new treatment normally do well because of an enhanced placebo effect, which is itself a function of the motivation, interest and enthusiasm of the pioneering doctors. The importance of the physician's attitude has been demonstrated in a number of conditions such as depression, and also in compliance with therapy.[28,32] Indeed one review concluded that 'most of the factors which influence compliance and non-compliance can be controlled to some extent by the doctor rather than the patient'.[32] The modern doctor tends to concentrate on evidence, getting the diagnosis and treatment right and providing his or her patient with the necessary information. It is quite an added burden to realise that he/she must also have a fundamental emotional impact on the patient in the surgery.

Expectation

Expectation is probably a prime factor in the placebo effect and several studies have shown that it can override any active effects of medication that we give. Placebo alcohol for instance, can produce effects that do not occur when alcohol itself is administered in disguised form.[37] Placebo alcohol can produce increased sexual arousal to erotic stimuli, increased aggressive behaviour and increased craving for consumption of alcohol.[38–41] The real thing in disguise, however, produces none of these effects! Expectancy can also have a negative effect on therapy. This has been shown in patients about to receive chemotherapy – around a quarter of whom vomit before actually receiving the treatment (the effect can be reversed by reversing the expectation through behavioural therapy).

If the average person thinks he/she is on a placebo, then the treatment does not work as well.[42] In a double-blind clinical trial to control obesity, patients were either given active drug (PPA) or a placebo. If they thought they were on active treatment (because they guessed that their appetite was being suppressed) then the patients were more likely to lose weight and have less difficulty dieting. Conversely, if they thought they were on placebo (guessed by lack of any side-effects) then they did not get these benefits. The guesses were sometimes right and sometimes wrong but what mattered was what the patients thought that they were taking rather than what they actually were taking. Again, we have an example where expectation is a more important factor than active therapy. Also the possibility that side-effects of treatment might themselves be an independent factor in improving the efficacy of a given treatment. We all have patients who believe that the nastier the treatment, the better the likely effect.

A study in general practice attempted to utilise the expectation effect in order to influence the clinical course of acute tonsillitis.[43] Fifty patients were given a standard consultation and the other 50 were given more detailed information about the diagnosis, treatment and prognosis of their disease with a more extensive physical examination than the control group. Two days later symptoms had significantly improved in the experimental group over the control group and significantly more of the experimental group felt that the treatment had helped them. Did the experimental group get better medicine or better healing? Another study showed that if anaesthetists spent more time talking to their patients prior to operation, then recovery was far quicker.[44] Again this may well be more a factor of the physician's caring and sympathetic attitude and his generosity with his time rather than what he actually said.

Patient expectation is, of course, not a fixed entity. The rapid change in expectation on the part of both patients and GPs in the last few years towards prescribing antibiotics shows how expectation can change. For physician healers, the art is not only to improve the placebo effect by recognising the expectation effect but also to make expectations more appropriate.

What sort of placebo?

While patients vary in their ability to respond to the placebo effect and doctors vary in their ability to encourage it – the nature of the placebo itself is an independent variable. What sorts of placebo are most effective? As many drug companies know, some shapes and colours of pills are more effective than others. Furthermore, the credibility of the treatment and the ritual that surrounds the way that it is given are also very important.[45] Operative intervention seems to have just about the most powerful placebo effect – ranging between an alarming 60% and 70%.[6,13] Interventions with an element of magic and mystery, such as TENS machines and ultrasound therapy, have their own added placebo effect – no doubt this applies for modern treatments such as laser therapy and MRI scans.[28,46] Placebos undoubtedly vary from culture to culture. For instance, the French use suppositories far more than the English, while the latter often appear to think that foul-tasting medicines are more likely to make them better.

Therapeutic setting

The placebo effect also depends upon where the treatment is offered.[47] Patients following cholecystectomy were assigned either to rooms looking on a 'natural scene' or rooms facing a brick building. The patients with a view through their window had shorter postoperative hospital stays, received fewer negative comments in nurses notebooks and took fewer potent analgesics than patients in the rooms facing the brick building. This is an interesting study, which should impact on the way that our surgeries look. Few waiting rooms have the 'don't do this, don't do that' that were the hallmark of laudable GP surgeries in the 1970s but do we design our surgeries to elevate our patients? For some patients, 'hospitals' can provide a therapeutically secure environment and this probably explains why patients with unbearable organic symptoms, as well as functional ones such as hyperventilation, often seem to miraculously improve once they have entered the hospital gates.

Severity of symptoms

Finally, does the severity of symptoms matter? For angina and pain at least, it seems that the more severe the symptoms the better the placebo effect. All the more so if these patients have a higher threshold for seeking help for their symptoms.[5,24,27] One might, therefore, expect that compliance would also be better if an illness is severe but this is not always so.[32] For instance, one study[48] showed that out of 90% of physically disabled patients who said that they would follow the doctor's orders, only 44% actually did so.

Summary

The majority of symptoms and diseases in primary care can be improved significantly simply through the placebo effect. The range of conditions includes, for instance, angina, congestive cardiac failure, hypertension, peptic ulcer disease, multiple sclerosis and dementia.

The strength of the placebo response depends partly on the patient, his/her personality attitudes, motivation and expectation, and partly upon the doctor. It also depends on the therapeutic setting, the type of treatment, the nature of the problem and its severity. We may have conventionally underestimated the placebo effect because the conditions under which it is most effective (e.g. organic illness in young psychologically normal patients) are exactly those in which we are least likely to give a placebo and where active medication is most likely to be given and credited for any beneficial effect.

If we wish to maximise the placebo effect then we must regard it as a complex process, which requires a very different set of skills from those conventionally taught in medical school.

References

1 Dixon M (1998) Does 'healing' benefit patients with chronic symptoms? A quasi-randomised trial in general practice. *J R Soc Med.* **91**: 183–8.

2 Harkness EF, Abbot NC, Ernst E (2000) Distant healing as a therapy for peripheral common warts; a randomised control trial. Submitted for publication.

3 Beecher HK (1955) The powerful placebo. *JAMA.* **159**: 1602–6.

4 Evans W, Hoyle C (1933) The comparative value of drugs used in continuous treatment of angina pectoris. *Q J Med.* **22**: 311–38.

5 Janicki AG, Orzechowska-Juzwenko K, Swiderska-Blonska T (1998) The methodological and clinical aspects of the placebo effect in angina pectoris. *Cor Et Vasa.* **30** (1): 35–42.

6 Dimond EG, Kittle CF, Crockett JE (1960) Comparison of internal mammary artery ligation and sham operation for angina pectoris. *Am J Cardiol.* **5**: 483–6.

7 Archer TP, Leier CV (1992) Placebo treatment in congestive heart failure. *Cardiol J.* **81** (2–3): 125–33.

8 Beutler JJ, Attevelt JT, Schouten SA *et al.* (1998) Paranormal healing and hypertension. *BMJ.* **296** (6635): 1491–4.

9   Balansard P, Baralla A, Gonzales T *et al.* (1987) Study of the placebo effect by the pressure profile method. *Presse Medicale – Paris.* **16** (1): 19–21.

10 Suchman AL, Ader R (1992) Classic conditioning and placebo effects in crossover studies. *Clin Pharmacol Ther.* **52** (4): 372–7.

11 Graham DY, Akdmar K, Dyck P *et al.* (1985) Healing of benign gastric ulcer: comparison of cimetidine and placebo in the united states. *Ann Inter Med.* **102** (5): 573–6.

12 Dobie RA, Sakai CS, Sullivan MD *et al.* (1993) Antidepressant treatment of tinnitus patients: report of a randomized clinical trial and clinical prediction of benefit. *Am J Otol.* **14** (1): 18–23.

13 Bretlau P, Thomsen J, Tos M, Johnsen NJ (1984) Placebo effect in surgery for Ménière's disease: a three year follow-up study of patients in a double blind placebo controlled study on endolymphatic sac shunt surgery. *Am J Otol.* **5** (6): 558–61.

14 Couch JR Jr (1987) Placebo effect and clinical trials in migraine therapy. *Neuroepidemiology.* **6** (4): 178–85.

15 Hirsch RL, Johnson KP, Camenga DL (1988) The placebo effect during a double blind trial of recombinant alpha 2 interferon in multiple sclerosis patients: immunological and clinical findings. *Int J Neurosci.* **39** (3–4): 189–96.

16 Spiegel D *et al.* (1989) Effect of psychosocial treatment on survival of patients with metastatic breast cancer. *Lancet.* **Oct 14**: 888–91.

17 Ratcliffe MA *et al.* (1995) Eysenck Personality Inventory L-scores in patients with Hodgkin's disease and non-Hodgkin's lymphoma. *Psychooncology.* **4**: 39–45.

18 Eccles M, Clarke J, Livingston M *et al.* (1998) North of England evidence-based guidelines in primary care management of dementia. *BMJ.* **317**: 802–8.

19 Medical Research Council (1965) Clinical trial of the treatment of depressive illness. *BMJ.* **I**: 881–6.

20 Raskin A *et al.* (1970) Differential response to chlorpromazine imipramine and placebo. *Arch Gen Psychiat.* **23**: 164–73.

21 Brown WA, Johnson MF, Chen MG (1992) Clinical features of depressed patients who do and do not improve with placebo. *Psychiat Res.* **41** (3): 203–14.

22 Morris PA (1982) The effect of pilgrimage on anxiety, depression and religious attitude. *Psychol Med.* **12** (2): 291–4.

23 Rosenberg NK, Mellergard M, Rosenberg R *et al.* (1991) Charac-teristics of panic disorder patients responding to placebo. *Acta Psychiat Scand* Suppl. **365**: 33–8.

24 Mavissakalian M (1988) The placebo effect in agraphobia – II. *J Nerv Ment Dis.* **176** (7): 446–8.

25 Meurice E (1986) Overall results of attempts to trear schizophre-nia by hemodialysis. Reflections on the placebo effect in a psychosis. *(French) Acta Psychiat Belg.* **86** (3): 266–86.

26 Mavissakalian MR, Jones B, Olson S (1990) Absence of placebo response in obsessive-compulsive disorder. *J Nerv Ment Dis.* **178** (4): 268–70.

27 Boureau F, Leizorovicz A, Caulin F (1988) The placebo effect in bone metastatic pain. *Presse Medicale – Paris.* **17** (21): 1063–6.

28 Hashish I, Hai HK, Harvey W *et al.* (1988) Reduction of post-operative pain and swelling by ultrasound treatment: a placebo effect. *Pain* **33** (3): 303–11.

29 Beecher HK, Keats AS, Mosteller F, Lasagna L (1953) The effect-iveness of oral analgesics (morphine, codeine, acetylsalicylic acid) and the problem of placebo 'reactors' and 'non-reactors'. *J Pharmacol Exp Ther.* **109**: 393–400.

30 White L, Tursky B, Schwartz GE (eds) (1985) *Placebo – Theory, research and mechanisms.* The Guildford Press, New York.

31 Long DM, Uematsu S, Kouba RB (1989) Placebo responses to medical device therapy for pain. *Stereotact Funct Neurosurg.* **53**: 149–56.

32 Evans L, Spelman M (1983) The problem of non-compliance with drug therapy. *Drugs* **25** (1): 63–76.

33 Balint M (1952) *The Doctor, The Patient and The Illness.* Pittman Medical, London.

34 Park LC, Covi L (1965) Non-blind placebo trial: an exploration of neurotic patients' responses to placebo when its inert content is exposed. *Arch Gen Psychiat.* **12**: 331–45.

35 Jensen MP, Karoly P (1991) Motivation and expectancy factors in symptom perception: a laboratory study of the placebo effect. *Psychosom Med.* **53** (2): 144–52.

36 Honigfeld G (1963) Physician and patient attitudes as factors infuencing the placebo response in depression. *Dis Nerv Syst.* **June**: 343–47.

37 Breckenridge RL, Dodd MO (1991) Locus of control and alcohol

placebo effects on performance in a driving simulator. *Percept Motor Skills.* **72** (3): 751–6.

38 Bridell DW, Rimm DC, Caddy GW *et al.* (1978) The effects of alcohol and cognitive set on sexual arousal to deviant stimuli. *J Abnorm Psychol.* **87**: 418–30.

39 Wilson GT, Lawson DM (1976) Expectancies, alcohol and sexual arousal in male social drinkers. *J Abnorm Psychol.* **85**: 587–94.

40 Lang AR, Goeckner DJ, Adesso J, Marlatt GA (1975) Effects of alcohol on aggression in male social drinkers. *J Abnorm Psychol.* **84**: 508–18.

41 Marlatt GA, Roshenow DJ (1991) Cognitive processes in alcohol use: expectancy and the balanced placebo design. In: NK Mello (ed.) *Advances in Substance Abuse.* J Kingsley, London.

42 Moscucci M, Byrne L, Weintraub M, Cox C (1987) Blinding, unblinding and the placebo effect: an analysis of patients' guesses of treatment assignment in a double-blind clinical trial. *Clin Pharmacol Ther.* **41** (3): 259–65.

43 Olsson B, Olsson B, Tibblin G (1989) Effect of patients' expectations on recovery from acute tonsillitis. *Family Pract.* 1989(Sep); **6** (3): 188–92.

44 Egbert LD, Battit GE, Welch CE, Bartlett MK (1964) Reduction of postoperative pain by encouragement and instruction of patients. *NEJM* **270**: 825–7.

45 Shapiro AK, Morris LA (1978) The placebo effect in medical and psychological therapies. In: SL Garfield, AE Bergin (eds) *Handbook of Psychotherapy and Behaviour Change.* John Wiley & Sons, New York.

46 Conn IG, Marshall AH, Yadav SN *et al.* (1986) Transcutanious electrical nerve stimulations following appendectomy: the placebo effect. *Ann R Coll Surg Engl.* **68** (4): 191.

47 Ulrich R (1984) View through a window may influence recovery from surgery. *Science.* **224**: 420–1.

48 Davis MS (1968) Variations in patients' compliance with doctors' orders: and empirical analysis of patterns of communication. *Am J Publ Health.* **58**: 274.

CHAPTER SEVEN

Why do placebos work?

We looked at *when* placebos work in the last chapter – this and the next chapter look at *why* and *how* they work. Armed with a credible theory and mechanism, the physician healer can be more confident, and consequently more effective, in his role.

There are two main theories as to why placebos work and these have a direct bearing on the efficacy of the physician healer.

Classical conditioning theory

Pavlov, the father of classical conditioning theory, was also the first to report a conditioned placebo effect when he observed that dogs showed morphine effects, whenever they were placed in an experimental chamber where they had previously received morphine. As we have seen, patients who do not initially respond to blood-pressure treatment with placebo can also be conditioned to respond to placebo following active treatment.[1]

Other experimental studies have also shown that the placebo response can be conditioned in humans. Lang and Rand[2] reported tachycardia in two out of three subjects when a conditioned placebo was substituted for glyceryl trinitrate. Other researchers have shown that the placebo response can be conditioned to a neutral cream following conditioning trials in which an analgesic cream was associated with pain reduction.[3] The basic model would maintain that neutral places (such as a doctor's surgery or the hospital), people (such as doctors or nurses), things (such as tablets, syringes or other medical instruments) and rituals (such as physical examinations, receiving an injection or taking medication) may be classically conditioned by association with previously experienced beneficial effects, which have occurred in these particular settings.[4] Clearly, conditioning is not limited to this environment and the patient will carry a number of other individual conditioned effects from his/her personal experiences, when he comes to surgery. Through 'response generalisation' the conditioned response will occur with treatments that are similar, although not necessarily identical, to the original one.

This theory has several important implications for general practice. First, in order to maintain a strong conditioned placebo effect, it is necessary that the therapeutic environment should be associated on a regular basis with effective treatment. This puts doctors and their surgeries rather than other therapists in by far the strongest position for maximising a placebo effect – simply because many orthodox treatments are so powerful and have proven effect. Furthermore, the theory would predict that doctors using powerful non-placebos and patients receiving them will tend to have an increased placebo effect. Those providing less effective medicines or who rely a lot on placebos will tend to have a lesser placebo effect. Hence, in chronic conditions, negative conditioned responses from previously ineffective therapy may generalise and the response of the patient to all treatments, whether active or placebo, will become correspondingly less. This phenomenon, whereby the response to placebo diminishes as increasing numbers of treatments fail, is called 'placebo sag'. It is probably a major factor in chronically ill 'heart sink' patients, who develop placebo sag to their treatments and their therapists. Such placebo sag may be specific to a particular GP and this could explain why the definition of 'heart sink' seems to depend upon the perception of the GP every bit as much as the external characteristics of the patient and why patients moving to another GP may often begin to thrive.

The theory also explains why so many patients insist that they improve on medications, which we as doctors feel cannot be effective. For instance, the patient given an 'inappropriate' antibiotic for a minor upper respiratory tract infection, who improves shortly afterwards (whether due to nature or the drug) will be conditioned to see his improvement as due to the antibiotic. Future prescription of the antibiotic will have both a symptomatic and possibly a physiological effect in improving his condition due to the conditioned placebo effect. Frequently, such prescriptions can become a 'folie â deux' with inappropriate, possibly harmful and expensive treatment being given to achieve only a placebo effect. This may explain why antibiotics have been traditionally over-prescribed and the challenge will be to exert a similar conditioned placebo effect but without giving the antibiotic.

GPs almost universally use placebos in some circumstances but tend to have negative feelings about doing so.[5] Conditioning theory would dictate that the frequent use of placebos by a doctor would make them increasingly ineffective and that the most effective way of maintaining a placebo effect is to give mainly active drugs. The ideal situation might be to condition a patient to an active drug, which will continue to give an effect equal to the original therapy because of the conditioned placebo response. In time, the patient would respond less well to the placebo than the original active drug but such reduction in effect could be prevented by using small amounts of non-placebo reinforcement from time to time. How might this look in practice? We know that a benign and gastric ulcer will be healed by a placebo in 45% of patients, which rises to 65% given a relatively old-fashioned treatment.[6] If we gave the active treatment with good effect to a patient on one occasion then the theory would be that a placebo form of this active medication on a subsequent occasion would give a placebo response higher than the average 45% placebo response. This might not seem ethical but it could explain why patients with various conditions can be maintained on diminishing amounts of medication because of a conditioned placebo effect (in addition to the active effect) when counter theories might predict that they should become physiologically habituated to a remedy and therefore need more of it to obtain a given effect.

Another consequence of this theory is that where 'placebo sag' has occurred with one sort of treatment (e.g. drugs), then a different method (e.g. injections, operations etc.) may become effective provided that placebo sag is not generalised to these methods of treatment as well. Alternatively, altering the context of treatment altogether by moving, for instance, to 'complementary therapy' may revive a placebo response that has previously atrophied in the conventional medical situation. The phenomenon of treatments that are effective for two or three months and then cease to be is commonly seen in general practice. It is probable that such treatments are only effective because of the placebo effect, which extinguishes predictably after two or three months.

A patient's responses are conditioned by his/her medical history and previous treatments and contact with medical services. The placebo response is thus individualistic, even idiosyncratic and becomes deeply rooted from a very early age. For instance, spoken messages in childrens books describe the doctor's conditioned response to give 'a medicine that will make you better', and this creates deep-rooted beliefs as to what should happen in medical encounters and what the outcome should be.[7] The second theory, concerning expectation, is simply an offshoot of classical conditioning theory.

The expectation effect

Faith, hope and belief are clearly important variables in producing a placebo effect and psychologists have conceptualised this in terms of 'cognitive expectancy', which assumes that a patient's specific expectation of improvement will be causally connected to the change that takes place.

We have already seen in studies on alcohol that the effects of a substance can depend more upon you expect to happen than what the substance actually contains. Laboratory studies have confirmed that expectation is an important factor in how you perceive your symptoms and the therapeutic outcome can depend more upon what you think you are taking than what you actually are taking.[8] We have also seen in a clinical situation how expectation can influence recovery from an acute condition.[9] Why should expectation work in this way? One theory is that if you expect a positive outcome then this gives illness an element of controllability. If you feel that you can control things then you will begin to feel better because you experience less stress, anxiety and feelings of helplessness. This may have physiological sequelae as well. It has also been suggested that positive expectation leads to more 'coping cognitions' or in layman's terms a more positive outlook, which can affect perception (e.g. of pain).

Wickramasekera,[4] who is a leading exponent of expectancy theory, listed the factors that can be used to enhance the placebo component of non-placebo treatment. These are:

- the credibility of the therapist
- the credibility of the therapeutic setting
- the credibility of the treatment per se
- the credibility of the administrative ritual and
- the nature of the interpersonal relationship between the patient and the therapist.

The emphasis then is on credibility – what doctors and patients know as 'trust. It is in order to maintain such credibility that most of us would think it unethical to knowingly use a placebo.

While psychological theory can tell us much about how we can improve the effectiveness of the placebo effect, biochemical and physiological explanations are beginning to tell us how it works. This is the subject of the next chapter.

Summary

The placebo effect is a conditioned response to improve. Improvement will occur when the patient comes across a set of conditions that have previously been associated with an improvement in his condition. Much of this may be unconscious, but positive expectation and belief that a treatment will work do seem to have an added effect. The consequence of this is that if a patient thinks that a treatment is likely to work then 'a priori' it is likely to do so. Conversely, if a patient does not believe that a treatment will work then some effort is required in order to explain why it might. Unless expectation is changed, the full effect of the treatment may not be realised.

References

1 Suchman AL, Ader R (1992) Classic conditioning and placebo effects in crossover studies. *Clin Pharmacol Ther.* **52** (4): 372–7.

2 Lang WJ, Rand MJ (1969) A placebo response as a conditional reflex to glyceryl trinitrate. *Med J Aust.* **1**: 912–14.

3 Voudouris NJ, Peck CL, Coleman G (1985) Conditioned placebo responses. *J Pers Soc Psychol.* **48**: 47–53.

4 Wickramasekera IA (1980) A conditioned response model of the placebo effect: predictions from the model. *Biofeedback Self Regul.* **5**: 5–18.

5 Thompson RJ, Buchanan WJ (1982) Placebos and general practice: attitudes to, and the use of, the placebo effect. *NZ Med J.* **95** (712): 492–4.

6 Graham DY, Akdmar K, Dyck P *et al.* (1985) Healing of benign gastric ulcer: comparison of cimetidine and placebo in the United States. *Ann Intern Med.* **102** (5): 573–6.

7 Banner A (1971) *Ant & Bee and The Doctor.* Kaye & Ward Ltd, London.

8 Jensen MP, Karoly P (1991) Motivation and expectancy factors in symptom perception: a laboratory study of the placebo effect. *Psychosom Med.* **53** (2): 144–52.

9 Olsson B, Olsson B, Tibblin G (1989) Effect of patients' expectations on recovery from acute tonsillitis. *Family Pract.* **6** (3): 188–92.

CHAPTER EIGHT

How does the placebo effect work? How can the mind affect the body? Evidence from psychoneuroimmunology

It is easy for the conventional doctor to understand that placebo may be a factor in altering a patient's *perception* of his disease and symptoms and thus improve them. Placebo effects, however, go far deeper than this and are not simply about the things seeming better but actually *being better*. This is why they should be part of mainstream medicine.

This area has been neglected in the past because we have been philosophically and physiologically unable to explain how mind can affect body. This is partly because we have separated them in the first place. Modern science, however, has provided ample evidence for a reintegration of mind and body both in theory and practice.

Effects of the mind upon the body

Almost every second of our lives we witness the effects of our mind and our bodies whether it be our mouths watering before a meal or our heart racing before an important event. Research has shown that a wide range of physiological responses can be conditioned including blood pressure, cardiac rate and rhythm, hormone levels, salivation, sweat secretion, immune response, bronchial airway resistance, respiration, ECG wave form and even blood glucose and skin temperature.

It is not surprising, therefore, that a wide range of psychological events should be constantly affecting our physical health. The stress-induced peptic ulcer or the increase in mortality following the death of a spouse are two examples of this common phenomenon.[1] Several studies have related the incidence of cancer to previous stress.[2] A recent study has demonstrated an important relationship between mental health and physical well-being in the prevention of heart disease.[3]

Few would doubt, therefore, that improving the individual or collective mental health of a community is likely to improve physical health as well. This fits nicely with the current developments of PCGs in the UK, which have given local healthcare professionals, particularly GPs, an extended role in the community outside traditional health boundaries. Thus the potential to improve the 'social capital' of the community in which they work may have an indirect effect upon physical health far in excess of previous campaigns that have been specifically directed only at the prevention of physical disease.

If the mind can lead to bad or good physical health can we use it to fight disease?

How can the mind heal the body?

Psychoneuroimmunology is beginning to explain a phenomenon that has been frequently observed by doctors and patients, but has previously been outside the remit of science.

The current theory is that the brain can reverse disease via a group of neurotransmitters called neuropeptides. These are triggered by the physiological equivalent of feelings and thoughts and can lock onto cells all over the body. Central transmitters of this kind may act directly on the body or indirectly via the endocrine and immunological systems.

A review article in the *New England Journal of Medicine*[4] concluded, 'a number of studies have shown that changes in systemic immune function occur after manipulations of the CNS, suggesting that immunocompetence can be regulated by the brain'. The brain can affect immune function and it can also affect hormones. The hypothalamus, for instance, is geographically close to and interconnected with the pituitary and is the brain's means of regulating endocrine activity. There are, however, lots of less predictable interconnections, as the hypothalamus also has a role in regulating humoral and cellular immunity, and it has been shown that lesions of the anterior hypothalamus can modify asthma.[5] The output of the brain can affect the body in this way and similarly feedback from the body to the brain can further regulate the body's response. Experimental destruction of the sensory enervation of joints has been shown to reduce the intensity of inflammatory arthritis, which suggests that the nervous system may also have a direct effect on the inflammatory process that is quite different from its effect on immunological markers.[6]

The brain may affect the body but this can work both ways. Endocrine activity can directly modify immunological function.[7] It seems likely that the flow of activity can go in the opposite direction as lymphocytes contain immunoreactive thyrotrophin and secrete corticotropin, growth hormone and prolactin.[8] Psychoneuroimmunology remains in its infancy but it is beginning to explain how the mind can affect the body. As it does so it is becoming clear that there are complex homeostatic, feedback and amplifying systems, which may one day be explained at a molecular level.

The immunological response to stress

Research on stress and relaxation has provided an interesting example of how these mechanisms might work. Stress generally has a negative action on the immune response. Activation of the sympathetic nervous system causes leucocytosis, lymphopenia and inhibition of natural killer cell activity.[9] It seems, however, that an animal under stress can improve its immunological profile if it is able to escape that stress. For instance, if a rat is unable to escape an electric shock then lymphocyte proliferation is suppressed, but this does not happen if it is able escape the shock.[10] Another study looked at the relationship between stress and developing cancer when rats were injected with tumour preparation. Those receiving escapable shocks were able to reject the tumour 63% of the time – much more than those who were not.[11,12] It is tempting to compare this work showing improved resistance and reduced metastases in a 'coping' mouse with the *Lancet* article already quoted, which showed the beneficial effects of psychosocial treatment on the survival of patients with metastatic breast cancer.[13]

Certainly, human research seems to confirm that stress depresses the immune system. Stress, for instance, increases susceptibility to infection via the common cold.[14] Conversely, social support (possibly as a 'de-stressor') can act as a buffer to a patient's vulnerability to infection.[15] Reduced activity of lymphocytes has been noted in bereaved spouses compared with controls.[16] A reduction in lymphoplast transformation in a group of psychiatry residents experiencing severe examination stress has also been noted.[17] Similarly lymphocyte production of interferon-γ and the activity of natural killer cells were reduced in medical students during examination time.[18] The same research has shown that you could reduce this decline in immune function by practising self-hypnosis. Indeed, a recent study has confirmed that such buffering of immune function with self-hypnosis does occur in terms of numbers of natural killer cells ($p<.002$) and increased cortisol levels.[19] Furthermore, the research has related these immunological improvements from hypnosis in examination students to improvement in mood and energy as well. So if you remove the stress, it seems that your immune profile will improve. This was found yet again in a study of homosexual men told that they were HIV negative, whose lymphocyte reactivity almost doubled within one week of the good news.[20]

The specific effects of stress on natural killer cell activity are particularly interesting. Natural killer cells kill viral-infected cells and also have antibacterial activity.[21,22] They are also thought to prevent the establishment of primary tumours, as well as limiting metastatic disease.[23] We have seen reduced activity in such cells with both animals and humans under stress.[9,18] Another study has confirmed this negative effect of stress/anxiety on natural killer cell activity and shown that depression also has a similar effect.[24] The same study showed that anger appeared to improve natural killer cell activity, which fits well with the improved immunological activity seen in mice who cope by fighting. It also fits with the common observation that people who fight their disease seem to do better and research, which shows that hostility in humans can improve the placebo response.[25]

If state of mind can affect killer cell activity – the crucial question is can we use the mind in order to increase our natural killer cell activity? A controlled study on 45 elderly people given one month's relaxation training showed a significant increase in natural killer cell activity, but which lasted for only one month.[26] A recent study showed that medical students trained in self-hypnosis before exams were able to significantly buffer the decline found in their fellow students because of the stressful situation. The students undertaking self-hypnosis also felt more energetic and calmer, and their degree of calmness was correlated with their killer cell (CD4) counts. The authors came to a conclusion that could have major implications for orthodox therapy, complementary therapy and indeed the way that we behave towards each other. 'The sizeable influences on immunity achieved by a relatively brief, low cost psychological intervention in the face of a compelling, but routine, stress in young, healthy adults have relevance to applications in the clinic and illness prevention.'[27]

Group therapy to reduce psychological distress in patients with a melanoma led, however, to a long-term (six months) improvement in both the numbers of different types of killer cell and their level of function.[24] The same researchers have also shown recently that this same intervention led to a significant increase in survival time.[28] Did increase in natural killer status lead to increase in survival time? The research did not show this but there was evidence that initial level of natural killer cell activity was related to later reoccurrence of the tumour. Nevertheless a recent study on 80 patients with locally advanced breast cancer showed that the more depressed patients were at the start of treatment (measured by the Hospital Anxiety and Depression scale), the poorer the response to primary chemotherapy $(p < .0001)$.[29] As depression is associated with reduced killer cell activity, the link between the state of mind, killer cells and therapeutic outcome in cancer begins to look firmer. This study also showed that relaxation training and creative visualisation led to a number of immunological improvements including activated killer cell cytotoxicity, which depended on the frequency of such treatment.

This path of research is becoming more interesting by the month. Previous studies, for instance, have linked reduced natural killer cell numbers with a tendency to recurrence of herpes simplex virus 1 and 2. A recent study has confirmed that hypnotherapy can increase natural killer cell numbers and actually reduce the number of recurrences of herpes simplex virus 1 and 2.[30] Furthermore, in this study only those who improved had increased numbers of killer cells suggesting that they might be an important part of the improved immunity to herpes simplex virus. Unpublished evidence (M Ghoneum, personal commun.) comparing Japanese communities from three different parts of the USA, who practice intensive self-healing (Johrei) with matched controls have demonstrated significant increases in the activity of killer cells in such communities. Observations of these same Johrei practitioners performing healing on each other (K Shiga, personal commun.) have shown an alteration in the pattern of EEG activity (alpha waves). In line with this, research from elsewhere has shown that electromagnetic stimulation of the brain (by transcranial magnetic stimulation) led to alterations in immune function.[31] Another study has shown that EEG patterns of HIV patients can predict immune competence two to three years later.[32]

Such research is now at a crossroads. In future it may be possible to associate alterations in the state of mind with changes in brain activity, immunological changes and therapeutic outcome. Operant conditioning of EEG patterns to improve the performance of singers is already being used. There are many tantalising therapeutic possibilities. For instance, it is well known that EEG patterns are abnormal in schizophrenia – could normalisation of these EEG patterns provide a way of curing or controlling schizophrenia? The possibilities seem endless. Nevertheless, it will be a long time before we can specify exactly what interactions between

GPs/therapist and his/her patient will lead to precisely what physiological changes and to quantify the therapeutic benefit that results.

It is also clear that the effects of stress depend very much on the type of stress and also on the nature of the person receiving the stress.[33,34] In the words of Professor John Gruzelier, who has performed much of this pioneering research at the Charing Cross and Westminster Medical School: 'What is stressful for one person is perceived as a challenge for another'. It seems that we are dealing with two types of stress. There is good stress where one can literally 'not afford to be ill' and bad stress, which depletes the activity and number of killer cells. In some ways the idea of good (escapable) stress and bad (inescapable) stress mirrors the concept of good (HDL) and bad (LDL) cholesterol. We can now explain why hypnosis and self-hypnosis are so effective – this is because they are able to change the patient's perception from bad stress to challenge. It also arms the physician healer with the hypothesis that he/she should not only mould his/her therapy to the patient's expectations, but should also alter those expectations where appropriate. The bottom line is that we cannot ignore the inevitability of there being psychoneuroimmunological effects in each and every consultation that we have with our patients. No conclusions can be made at this stage but it is tempting to hypothesise that the interaction between therapist/GP and patient might lead to an alteration in brainwave activity, which itself may affect output of transmitter substances, hormones and immunological cells.

Pain response

Pain has also been well researched in humans, where it is now thought that the placebo effect may be mediated largely by the activation of endogenous opiates. This hypothesis has been partially confirmed by research suggesting that the analgesia produced by placebo was partially reversible with naloxone.[35] To date three studies have shown that pain relief generated by placebo can be reversed by naloxone, while two studies have failed to show this effect. The differing results of these studies are probably explained by different methodologies, types of pain and different patient states in all the studies.

The plausible conclusion is that some placebo pain relief is via endogenous opiates and some via non-opioid mechanisms.[36] Specific non-opiate receptors for beta-endorphin have, for instance, been discovered.[37] The pain pathways interact with the immunological system in very much the same way as we have seen the neurological and immune systems interacting elsewhere. This may be why, for instance, morphine receptors have been found on normal human blood T lymphocytes.[38]

Training the immune system

If our theories see the placebo effect as a conditioned reflex – is there any evidence that the immunological system can itself be conditioned? It seems that it can. Studies on grafts have confirmed that conditioned suppression can occur at both humoral and cellular levels of the immune system. Ader et al.[39] showed a similar effect in mice with autoimmune disease. They were later able to demonstrate the clinical importance of these cellular changes in mice with systemic lupus erythematosus (SLE) syndrome, which can normally be controlled using immunosuppressive drugs. He found that by pairing normal saccharin with immunosuppressant injections he could build up a conditioned response whereby saccharin alone was later able to suppress the SLE syndrome. These results, which were both clinically and statistically significant, provide an elegant demonstration of how a psychological association might lead to an altered immunological effect.

Summary

Few would doubt that our state of mind has a major bearing upon our state of health. It is surprising, therefore, that there has been little effort to improve the mental health of communities compared with efforts aimed specifically at preventing physical disease. Few would also doubt that our mental state can also effect our perception of disease. The main question, however, is to what extent can the mind actually bring about physiological changes that cure or improve disease? Psychoneuroimmunology is now advanced enough to tell us how this might happen and provide one or two examples of how this does happen. Increasingly, it seems that we will one day be able to link the 'human' intervention with alterations in the brainwaves and immuno-competence and symptoms of our patients. Armed with such knowledge we will be able to use ourselves as therapists to bring about such changes – backed by biotechnical medicine when appropriate.

In terms of providing clinically useful predictions for any given intervention, however, we are still at an early stage.

Conclusions

The implications of placebo research

The placebo effect is the strongest, the most comprehensive and the most proven medicine available to GPs. A proper understanding of the placebo effect in our patients could greatly improve our therapeutic effect and reduce the cost of medicines and procedures. Why, therefore, has the placebo effect been so ignored?

One answer is that it has not been very much researched. Much of our knowledge about the placebo effect is incidental as funding (particularly from pharmaceutical companies) for placebo research is difficult to obtain. This seems odd, particularly in the UK, where the state-run service would have everything to gain from greater knowledge about it. Another reason why it has been underestimated is that placebos, when they are given, are probably given to the least appropriate patients – the neurotic, the heart sink and the chronically ill (with placebo sag). These are the occasions when placebos are least likely to work.

We also probably try to judge the size of the placebo effect by seeing how well a treatment, which we do not particularly believe in, works for the patient. When it fails to work we say to ourselves: 'That is because this is not an effective treatment and when a treatment is not effective the patient does not respond to it – so any placebo effect is minimal'. Yet, as we know the placebo effect will be minimal if the doctor does not believe that a treatment is effective in the first place.

Conversely, when we are most enthusiastic in our belief in a particular drug, which works wonderfully, we ascribe all that effect to the active drug, omitting to realise that these are precisely the circumstances when we ourselves exert a maximum placebo effect. The belief of the modern doctor in his medicine thus becomes a self-fulfilling prophecy. In a sense he has to ignore the placebo effect because when he admits to himself that a drug might not work then its placebo effectiveness is reduced as well.

This is why it is so interesting to study the effectiveness of discredited treatments prior to their recognition as being ineffective. It also makes one wonder how many treatments, which we swear by now, will be laughed at in a 100 years time. One suspects that every generation of doctors have had far too much faith in their medicines and procedures and thus underestimated (though paradoxically accentuated) the placebo effect in their therapeutic regimes.

Another reason why we have underestimated the placebo effect is because we have failed to analyse what it is or to see it as a variable effect, which depends very much upon our own performance. It is necessary to distinguish (in theory at least) the degree of natural recovery that might occur when a patient is given a placebo, the extra effect when that placebo is given in an average medical consultation and the added effect that can be obtained from trying to maximise the placebo effect in such a consultation. If any study in medicine should be carried out, it is this one. The point is that when we say that medication has an average of 35% placebo effect, we ignore the much better effects that might be obtained in certain situations with certain diseases.[40] A double-blind, cross-over study will give only a minimal placebo effect. A retrospective study of treatment that was once thought to be generally effective will tend to be nearer what happens in real life. If GPs thought that the actual placebo effect was far higher than the normally quoted to 35%, as it undoubtedly is, then we would all have taken it much more seriously. Particularly as the effect very much depends upon how we use it.

While undermining the placebo effect we have been more than happy to overrate the effect of our treatments. We rush to prescribe something that shows a statistically significant improvement over a placebo, but rarely enquire as to whether this difference is clinically significant enough to merit giving the active treatment. For instance, the trial already quoted on gastric ulceration showed a healing rate at six weeks of 45% on placebo and 65% on Cimetidine.[40] Mathematically this would suggest that 70% of the effects of Cimetidine are due to placebo (although the logic of saying this is questionable). If this is so, why have we not been researching furiously to detect those categories of patients for whom the active treatment provides no significant improvement over the placebo treatment? The answer is that we have had no motive to do so. Nor, perhaps, are we intellectually honest with ourselves. If 39% of patients respond to placebos given for depression after four weeks and if 68% of patients have stopped their active medication within this time and without their GP's knowing then it is very questionable how effective most of our 'active' medication can be.[41,42] Yet these are facts that we choose to ignore in favour of the results of double-blind and cross-over studies.

What we should really be looking at is the power and generality of the placebo response. Placebo research is beginning to tell us that the placebo effect is far greater than we might have previously believed and that this power can be explained by looking at our psychological and physiological makeup. The strength of placebo research is that it highlights the very important role of the minds of both doctor and patient in improving physical health. The weakness is that it emphasises the doctor's role in the context of giving placebos and probably underestimates his role in the context of a consultation where either an active medication or no medication at all is given. In such consultations the placebo effect is largely invisible. Nevertheless, placebo research provides many suggestions that will be taken up in future chapters, when looking specifically at how we might change our therapeutic practice.

In 1952 Michael Balint proposed the question 'why do placebos sometimes achieve what we expect from them, sometimes astonish us by achieving much more, and sometimes fail us painfully?' He added, 'we must point to the need for more and properly planned research, as any real understanding of these problems would certainly profoundly influence the nation's health, high drug bill and unnecessarily overworked specialist services'. In the words of one group of researchers 'if we continue to ignore the placebo effect and the minds of our patients, it is no longer simply a matter of lacking courtesy, but it is also a scientific error'.[43] These comments seem embarrassingly reasonable but we have done little about them so far. The fundamental reason, outlined at the beginning of this book, is that we have been obsessed with technological medicine and an evidence base that has largely depended upon secondary care research. The worm is turning and a primary care-led NHS should lead to a new confidence in what primary care is offering and a realisation that what we are offering is more than a soup kitchen for evidence-based medicine. What we now need is a far greater evidence base that will unlock the secrets of the effective physician healer.

References

1   Stein M, Miller AH, Trestman RL (1991) Depression, the immune system, and health and illness. *Arch Gen Psychiat*. **48**: 171–7.

2   Anisman H, Sklar LS (1985) Stress as a moderator variable in neoplasia in Tursky and Schwartz. *Placebo*. 356.

3   Kawachi I, Colditz GA *et al.* (1996) A prospective study of social networks in relation to total mortality and cardiovascular disease in men in the U.S.A. *J Epidemiol Community Health*. **50**: 245–51.

4   Reichlin S (1993) Neuroendocrine–immune interactions. *NEJM*. **Oct 21**: 1247.

5   Mrazek DA, Klinnert M (1991) Asthma: psychoneuroimmunologic considerations In: R Ader, DL Felton, N Cohen (eds) *Psychoneuroimmunology* (2e). Academic Press, San Diego, CA.

6   Kidd BL, Mapp PI, Gibson SJ *et al.* (1989) A neurogenic mechanism for symmetrical arthritis. *Lancet* **2**: 1128–30.

7   Ader R, Felten DL, Cohen N (eds) (1991) *Psychoneuroimmunology* (2e). Academic Press, San Diego, CA.

8   Kelley KW, Arkins S, Li YM (1992) Growth hormone, prolactin, and insulin-like growth factors: new jobs for old players. *Brain Behav Immun*. **6**: 317–657.

9   Weiss JM, Sundar S (1992) Effects of stress on cellular immune responses in animals. *Rev Psychiat*. **11**: 145–80.

10 Laudenslager ML (1993) Coping and immunosuppression: inescapable but not escapable shock suppresses lymphocyte proliferation. *Science*. **221**: 568–70.

11 Visintainer MA, Volpicelli JR, Seligman MEP (1982) Tumor rejection in rats after inescapable or escapable shock. *Science*. **216**: 437–39.

12 Sklar LS, Anisman H (1979) Stress and coping factors influence tumor growth. *Science*. **205**: 513–15.

13 Spiegel D *et al.* (1989) Effect of psychosocial treatment on survival of patients with metastatic breast cancer. *Lancet.* **Oct 14**: 888–91.

14 Cohen S, Doyle WJ, Skoner DP *et al.* (1997) Social ties and susceptibility to the common cold. *JAMA.* **277** (24):1940–4.

15 Cohen S, Wills TA (1985) Stress, social support and the buffering hypothesis. *Psychol Bull.* **98**: 310–57.

16 Bartrop RW, Luckhurst E, Lazarus L *et al.* (1977) Depressed lymphocyte function after bereavement. *Lancet.* **1–11**: 834–6.

17 Dorian BJ, Keystone E, Garfinkel PE, Brown GM (1981) Immune mechanisms in acute psychological stress. *Psychosom Med.* **43**: 84 (abstracts).

18 Keicolt-Glaser JK, Glaser R (1991) Stress and immune function in humans. In: R Ader, DL Felton, N Cohen (eds) *Psychoneuroimmunology* (2e). Academic Press, San Diego, CA.

19 Gruzelier J *et al.* (2000) Prophylactic benefits of hypnosis on cell mediated immunity and cortisol during exam stress. Submitted for publication.

20 Antoni MH, Schneiderman N, Klimas N *et al.* (1991) Disparities in psychological, neuroendocrine and immunologic patterns in asymptomatic HIV-1 seropositive and seronegative gay men. *Biol Psychiat.* **29**: 1023–41.

21 Biron CA, Natuk RJ, Welsh RM (1986) Generation of large granular T lymphocytes *in vivo* during viral infection. *J Immunol.* **136**: 2280–6.

22 Garcia-Penarrubia P, Koster FT, Kelley RU *et al.* (1989) Anti bacterial activity of natural killer cells. *J Exp Med.* **169**: 99–113.

23 Richards SJ, Scott CS (1992) Human natural killer cells in health and disease. *Leukaemia Lymphoma.* **7**: 377–99.

24 Fawzy FI, Kemeny ME, Fawzy NW *et al.* (1990) A structured psychiatric intervention for cancer patients. II. Changes over time in immunological measures. *Arch Gen Psychiat.* **47**: 729–35.

25 Raskin A *et al.* (1970) Differential response to chlorpromazine, imipramine and placebo. *Arch Gen Psychiat.* **23**: 164–73.

26 Kiecolt-Glaser JK, Glaser R, Williger D *et al.* (1985)Psychosocial enhancement of immunocompetence in a geriatric population. *Health Psychol.* **4**: 25–41.

27 Gruzelier J, Smith F, Nagy A *et al.* (2000) Prophylactic benefits at exam time on cell medicated immunity through self hypnosis training. Submitted for publication.

28 Fawzy FI, Fawzy NW, Hyun CS *et al.* (1993) Malignant melanoma: effects of an early structured psychiatric intervention coping, and affective state on recurrence and survival 6 years later. *Arch Gen Psychiat.* **50**: 681.

29 Walker LG *et al.* (1997) Psychological factors predict response to neoadjuvant chemotherapy in women with locally advanced breast cancer. *Br J Surg.* **84** (Suppl. 1): 46.

30 Fox PA, Henderson DC, Barton SE *et al.* (2000) Immunological markers of frequently recurrent genital herpes simplex virus and their response to hypnotherapy. Submitted for publication.

31 Clow A *et al.* (2000) Direct evidence for corltical regulation of immune and glucocorticoid function in healthy conscious humans. Submitted for publication.

32 Gruzelier J *et al.* (1996) Prospective associations between lateralised brain function and immune status in HIV infection: analysis of EEG, cognition and mood over 30 months. *Int J Psychphysiol.* **23**: 215–24.

33 Evans P *et al.* (1997) Stress and the iummune system. *Psychologist.* **10**: 303–7.

34 Lazar I (2000) Psychoimmunoligcal and autonomic consequences of impending unemployment. Submitted for publication.

35 Posner J, Burke CA (1985) The effects of naloxone on opiate and placebo analgesia in healthy volunteers. *Psychopharmacology.* **87**: 468–72.

36 Peck C, Coleman G (1992) Implications of placebo theory for clinical research and practice in pain management. *Theoretical Med.* **12**: 247–70.

37 Hazum E, Chang KJ, Cuatrecasas P (1979) Specific non-opiate receptors for beta-endorphin. *Science.* **205**: 1033–5.

38 Wybran J, Appelboom T, Famaey J, Gouvaerts A (1979) Suggestive evidence for receptors for morphine and methionine-enkephalin on normal human blood T lymphocytes. *J Immunol.* **123**: 1068–70.

39 Ader R, Grota LJ, Cohen N (1987) Conditioning phenomena and immune function. *Ann NY Acad Sci.* **496**: 532–44.

40 Beecher HK (1955) The powerful placebo. *JAMA.* **159**: 1602–6.

41 Graham DY, Akdmar K, Dyck P *et al.* (1985) Healing of benign gastric ulcer: comparison of cimetidine and placebo in the united states. *Ann Intern Med.* **102** (5): 573–6.

42 Medical Research Council (1965) Clinical trial of the treatment of depressive illness. *BMJ*. 881–6.

43 Johnson DAW (1973) Treatment of depression in general practice. *BMJ*. **2**: 18.

CHAPTER NINE

How the physician healer works: three theories

The evidence given so far should now help us to make a stab at explaining how and why the physician healer works for his/her patients. The important thing to remember is that the end result is not something that the physician healer does to the patient but something that the patient ultimately does to him/herself – a self-healing process generated by the efforts of the physician healer. It is an art that has to be very specific to the preconceptions and makeup of the patient him/herself. Generalisations are fine so far as they go, but they will not do in the treatment of the individual patient.

The three theories presented look at the physician healer role in three different respects. The first in terms of the process of the consultation, the second in terms of the different levels of relationship between therapist and patient, the third looks at the economic implications of the physician healer. They are designed to provide a perspective on the workings of the physician healer and not to be comprehensive or exclusive.

Theory A: How does the physician healer work?

Theory A postulates a cascade effect, which starts with the germ of a feeling that improvement is both desirable and possible, and ends mainly through altered perception with an improved physical state. The crucial element in any consultation is that the doctor should be able to 'throw the switch' that transfers the patient from one who is borne down by disease to one that can begin to conquer it. Some of our patients are on the threshold of such change when they come to see us and the task is easy for the physician healer. Others are far from this stage and tiring work, often lasting many consultations, or a change in life circumstances may be necessary before we can bring about the change that allows self-healing to begin. Figure 9.1 on p. 96 shows how a patient progresses during therapy from a position of 'I want to get better' to 'I am better'.

Pre-consultation

At the beginning, most patients will want to get better and this desire will both pre-date and initiate the consultation. In a few, where there is no real desire to get better, the healing process is likely to be blocked. This may occur, for instance, in cases where there is litigation involved or secondary gain.

Given that he/she wants to get better, the likelihood is that the patient will choose a port of call that he/she thinks will make him/her better depending upon both his/her own and received opinions. Thus seeing the GP at all is a positive decision made in the expectation of a positive response and outcome. The degree of expectation and compliance of treatment will be greater if the patient has a good personal relationship with the doctor that he/she sees. Quite frequently, the patient may begin to feel better prior to the consultation – in part because of his/her confidence in what the consultation may bring about. Hence the frequent refrain 'I always feel better by the time I see you, doctor'.

Consultation

The patient's preconceptions about the consultation itself may lead to improvement regardless of what actually happens in the consultation. This explains the observation made earlier in this book that patients sitting one side of a screen behind which they think is a spiritual healer (when there is not) may make a remarkable recovery. The patient following a medical consultation may similarly be affected by a conditioned response that tells him/her that once the consultation is over things will start to improve. There will be a sense of relief that the wait for the consultation and diagnosis is over, that the doctor and patient have finished their work and he/she can now relax and wait for the cure to start in the knowledge that nothing further needs to be done.

Thus the process of 'having a consultation' is itself therapeutical though the actual content of that consultation is also clearly a vital factor. Part Three of this book explores how we might improve the therapeutic content of each consultation in practice. Nevertheless, the end result should be that the patient is more relaxed and less fearful of his/her condition having been given some explanation and reassurance about his/her symptoms – possibly because he now sees them as fitting a pattern and amenable to some sort of control either by him/herself or the doctor. If it has been a positive and warm consultation, the patient should be in a more positive emotional state and emerge feeling more confident and better about him/herself in general. Previous chapters on placebo research have already shown us the importance of reducing stress, improving emotional state and offering 'escape options'. These will have a positive effect not only on the patient's perception of his/her physical state but also on the physical state itself.

Thus hopefully the patient leaves the consultation feeling slightly better in him/herself and/or hopeful that things will improve. Sometimes this process can be so effective that the patient will volunteer remarks prior to leaving such as: 'I am feeling better already'.

Post-consultation

Once the patient leaves the surgery, the 'cascade effect' starts as a factor of the patient's altered perception and behaviour following the consultation. With a more positive frame of mind towards his/her symptoms and their future improvement, the patient will begin to selectively attend to things that show progress and improvement and attend less to negative aspects of his/her situation. Chance or equivocal occurrences will be interpreted with a positive bias and the more good effects that are seen the more the patient will condition him/herself to expect and perceive more. Inevitably, this altered perception will translate itself into altered behaviour and the patient will perceive that he/she is able to do more, is less handicapped and therefore in time begin to do more. As he/she overcomes the barriers imposed by these symptoms, he/she will feel more in control and become master rather than victim of those symptoms.

As the patient does more, by a process of simple distraction, he/she will have less time to notice and be concerned about his/her previous symptoms. Thus, for instance, when he/she is exposed to previously fearful or painful events, he/she will find that he/she can deal with them better and this in itself will lead to behavioural reinforcement and partial extinction of the fear or pain. This altered self-perception will be mirrored by an altered perception of the patient by others, who will reinforce his/her own perception that he/she is improving. This more positive attitude will also make the patient more positive towards any active treatment that is offered (e.g. his/her compliance will improve). This will clearly increase the patient's exposure to the hopefully beneficial effects of active treatment, but we also know that improved compliance is also independently related to improved morbidity and mortality.[1]

In this way, small changes seen at the end of the consultation lead through this cascade effect to a vastly amplified healing effect, where the patient actually begins to feel better altogether. It may explain why patients will often say that they are already feeling better only half an hour after taking an antibiotic. It is likely that the placebo or healing effect will be much greater when active treatment is given rather than a simple placebo. The reason for this now becomes apparent. When the patient on active medication receives an unambiguous impression that the medication is affecting one or more of his/her symptoms, then the amplified healing effects due to altered perception and behaviour will be far greater than when he/she has to rely on a hunch that things might be improving. Indeed this may be so, to a lesser extent, if he/she is only experiencing recognised side-effects of treatment, which will confirm the power of what the patient is taking. Reverse logic may explain why the side-effects of placebos are frequently greater than those of active treatment.

Both conditioning and expectancy theory would predict the cascade effect: that is to say the patient that is feeling slightly better will be expected via positive reinforcement and increased expectation to get better still. On a physiological level, the cascade effect can be seen in terms of positive feedback. The psychological effects of the healing process are mirrored by increased neurotransmitter output affecting, for instance, endocrine and immunological systems. Changes in these systems feedback to central and peripheral neurotransmitter receptors, and thereby amplify further any neurotransmitter output.

For some patients (e.g. migraine sufferers) the continuum from 'I am feeling better' to 'I am better' is probably academic. For others (e.g. those with atopic eczema) any improvement in symptoms is likely to be reflected in an improvement in the visible physical condition. Where the symptoms are due to physiologically reversible disease, then the changes in symptoms, perception, attitude and behaviour are likely to lead to an improvement in the underlying physical process itself. Nevertheless, it would be unwise to overstate the case. For instance, anatomical problems such as hernias and varicose veins are unlikely to fit this model. Cancers too may frequently have progressed to a stage where they cannot be reversed by the processes discussed, although it seems that life expectancy can be improved.[2–4]

Finally, it would be unwise to suggest that the physician healer can frequently work this magic through one consultation. As we know from psychotherapy, an altered psychological state may come only after many months of treatment and sometimes after treatment has finished. Physical benefits, seen in reversible physiological processes, may come sometime after the psychological change that brought them about. The speed of the process will depend to some extent upon the patient's own psychological development and the size of effect will depend upon the reversibility of the disease process itself.

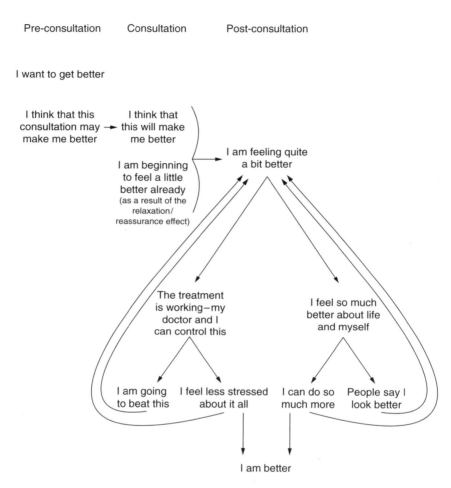

Figure 9.1: The nature of a possible cascade effect when the physician healer is successful.

Theory B: The different roles of the physician healer

This theory looks not at the process of healing, but more at the different roles of the physician healer. These are summarised in Figure 9.2.

1 Diagnosis and conventional treatment

2 Passive healing

3 Active healing

4 Director

Figure 9.2: The doctor as healer.

Diagnosis and conventional treatment

Explicitly, many patients come to a doctor to receive (and many doctors feel that their job is to give) a diagnosis and orthodox medical treatment. The skill of the physician healer will be to know when this is all that is appropriate and not to over-complicate the issue. He will also need to weed out those patients who do not want to lose their symptoms and who may be as immune to any therapeutic intervention by the GP as they have been previously to active medical treatments themselves.

Passive healing

The doctor who provides passive healing to his patients is maintaining the traditional doctor–patient relationship with the doctor himself being regarded as the healer. He is, of course, no more than a catalyst for self-healing, but this is not explicitly recognised within the relationship. As passive healer the doctor will have all the qualitites of a good pastoral doctor being able to comfort, support, reassure and empathise with his/her patients. Although passive healing is effective – the effect as with passive immunisation is likely to be temporary. The patient will return to the doctor for his 'fix'. For this reason doctors who are good at passive healing have been accused of encouraging dependency in their patients. All the same it is equally inappropriate to reject this role when patients are unable or unready to consider the doctor in the role of active healer.

Active healing

This represents progression in the relationship between patient and doctor from the straightforward passive/active role. The aim is to encourage patients to see that they themselves, rather than the doctor, are the 'agents of change'. No longer 'victims' but people who can cope with the problems themselves. The patient starts to feel he/she is in control and thus able, when necessary, to activate an innate self-healing capacity him/herself. This creates changes in behaviour, which not only help presenting problems but also stop problems being created and thus prevent disease. The final aim, of course, is self-dependence in which the patient feels able to seek the answer to his/her problems within him/herself rather than relying on the doctor for support and direction. Psychoneuroimmunology would seem to support this aim. If a patient is visualised as a sea of therapeutic substances (e.g. endorphins, antibodies, hormones and neuropeptides) and pathways – then he/she is the one best placed to pull the switches that control their release.

This new found capacity of the patient to heal him/herself should be seen as a liberating influence, which not only de-professionalises the whole process of getting better, but it also puts the doctor in his/her right place rather than on a pedestal. The patient may begin to realise the value of his/her therapeutic encounters with non-professionals – particularly friends and relatives who may have as important (if not more so) a therapeutic role in their lives as the professional.

Director

In the advanced relationship between doctor and patient the doctor becomes a director rather than dictator of healthcare. The relationship between doctor and patient has now changed from that of the patient as child, as seen at the passive healing stage, to that of adult. The patient is now able to activate his innate self-healing capacity, but still requires the doctor for information, technical help and, where appropriate, as counsellor. Such a relationship may be attainable in only a few patients, but the attempt is justified in most. A similar aim is echoed by Ivan Illich: 'Better healthcare will not depend on some new therapeutic achievement, but on the willingness of people to engage in self care'.

Which role and when?

Doctors need to be flexible as to which role of physician/healer they adopt. In order to control their symptoms and diseases, patients need to feel that they are under someone's control. Ideally, as we have seen, this is their own control, but failing that the doctor must offer him/herself as controller. This is his/her role as passive doctor/healer and a substantial number of patients will only able to relate to him/her in this role. Other patients, who are normally more active in their own treatment, may at times require a passive doctor/healer relationship when they are under extreme stress or are faced with very serious illnesses. For such people under such circumstances, the doctor is bound to offer him/herself as passive doctor/healer. To try and push the patient into a more active mode, when it is not appropriate can only be interpreted as not caring.

It is equally wrong to hold back the patient who is looking for a more active relationship with his/her doctor. This is sometimes frustrating and even frightening for the traditional doctor but if a patient wants control then it should be encouraged. All the evidence suggests that he/she will do better if he/she is given it. All the more so when it is apparent to the patient that the doctor has not got any control of his/her disease. In this situation the doctor may obstruct his/her patient's progression towards self-dependence because he/she may feel that it shows up his/her own inadequacy, but to do so only leads to a dysfunctional unhappy relationship between patient and doctor. The different roles of doctor/healer are also relevant in health promotion. For instance, mild coercion rather than neutral information may be more effective in the passive relationship, whereas the reverse would be true in a more active form of relationship.

There is a paradox in all this. We have said many times in this book that modern medicine must call back the physician healer if it is to improve its effectiveness. Yet in the most advanced relationship between doctor and patient, the patient has him/herself effectively taken on the role of physician healer and requires the doctor only as medical expert and advisor. So the effective physician healer eventually makes him/herself redundant and empowers the patient in this role. Thus, effectively, the ideal therapeutic solution is the patient as healer.

The patient as healer

The medical dictum 'do one, see one, teach one' should apply to patients every bit as much as to doctors. The patient who has progressed through the stages outlined should be able to heal other patients him/herself. Indeed their better knowledge of what it feels like to be a patient should put them in a better position to heal others. We should not underestimate the ability of patients to catalyse healing in each other independent of the medical context, and should encourage and empower them to do so. Societies that encourage individuals to look after each other and in particular to exert their powers of healing in whatever shape or manner on each other, should flourish. The new primary care-led NHS with PCGs should be in exactly this sort of position to raise the 'social capital' of their localities. Such a vision may seem threatening to many doctors who might fear that they would be asked to take a back seat in any revolution of this sort. They should be reassured that if they can encourage such a process then they will be rewarded with better resources for conventional medicine, when it is appropriate and more receptive patients when they see them.

Conclusion

The problem is that our personality types tend to make us either the supportive doctor or the doctor who fosters independence. The doctor who encourages and enables a whole locality to help itself independent of the medical context will require another personality type still. Successful therapists will be able to alternate between all three depending upon the context and presenting problem and patient. Nevertheless, to perceive the correct role required either by intuition or negotiation and then to move the consultation into that correct mode presents a considerable challenge to the most experienced GP. The Holy Grail of catalysing not only a patient, but the whole locality towards self-healing presents yet a further challenge. If, however, the emphasis is to move from the disease to preventing illness and finally to restoring and maintaining health then this is a challenge that must be met. Aneurin Bevan's hope that the NHS would improve health and thereby reduce costs was never realised. This is partly because we were locked in our surgeries and neither saw ourselves as responsible for the health of a whole locality nor provided it with the therapeutic know-how to maintain health. It was hardly the fault of GPs as the system discouraged them from going beyond the consulting room. Recent changes in the NHS, however, will emphasise the role of health promotion and improving the environment. For GPs, a belief in the self-healing capacity of our patients and an ability to help them to pass this knowledge on to each other will be vital factors if Bevan's ideal is to ever be realised. It is no coincidence that complementary therapies are so popular at present and research shows that their common thread is the promotion of self-healing.[5]

Theory C: Economic theory

From what has been said we can identify at least three ther-apeutic aspects for any given treatment over and above spon-taneous remission. These are:

- the active effect of a drug or procedure
- the intrinsic placebo effect of any given drug or procedure – this is a constant, for instance, in any double-blind placebo-controlled trial and suggests that there is 30% placebo effect for a wide range of treatments
- the therapeutic effect of the doctor.

When we say that a discredited treatment had a 50–60% placebo effect in its time, we are saying that the whole culture in which it was given almost doubled the standard placebo effect that might have been expected. Clearly, also this is only an average effect in either case and will be largely variable from therapist to therapist and undoubtably it will vary for any one therapist at different times.

Figure 9.3 shows the relative importance of these three effects over time. Prior to point X on the graph (around the turn of the century), most drugs had little therapeutic effect and successful treatment depended largely on the intrinsic placebo effect of any given drug or procedure plus any added effect that the doctor was able to produce in the therapeutic encounter. Between points X and Y (1900–2000) there has been a phase of rapid technological development and placebo/therapeutic effects have been dwarfed by the rapidly increasing efficacy of technical medicine. Beyond point Y there is a significant fall off in this rapid improvement produced by new medical developments because they are inap-propriate or ineffective in dealing with the remaining presenting problems, their marginal beneficial effect gets smaller or some of the technology becomes unaffordable. It is at this point Y, where general practice stands today, that it makes sense to improve the therapeutic efficiency of the doctor/patient encounter in purely cost/economic terms rather than to plough ever greater amounts into technology. Effectively, if we can improve our success as physician healers the whole curve moves upwards at point Y to Y_0 and this is not only a cost-effective way of improving

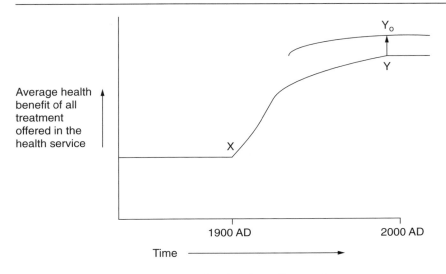

Figure 9.3: Improvements in health benefits with time.

therapeutic outcome, but it also represents a way of saving money for the technology that we can afford.

Figure 9.4 looks at the same question in monetary terms. If you spend no money on drugs or technology then all the therapeutic effects of your health service will be due to placebo and placebo effects. As you start putting money into the system between points P and Q your cost-effective medicines and procedures will be the major determinants of health gain. After point Q, the gains in any health spending on medicines and procedures starts to become marginal as new technology becomes increasingly expensive with relatively small gains as far as the health of the general population is concerned. As in Figure 9.3, it is at point Q that the variable added therapeutic effect of the encounter between patient and doctor becomes a significant force again. At this point increasing the efficiency of the physician healer will lead to greater health gain than further investment in technological medicine and once again money can be spared for when technological medicine really is needed.

It is not possible to quantify these effects at this stage. We know that the 'fixed intrinsic placebo effect' of any medication is around 30–35%, when a medicine is inactive. We do not know the size of this effect when an active medicine is given and there

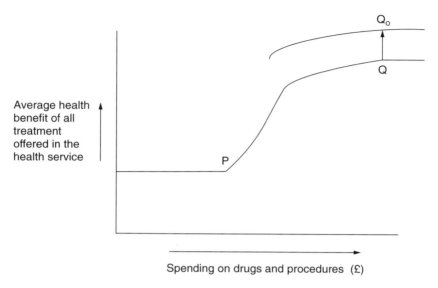

Figure 9.4: Improvements in health benefits with expenditure.

will be many variables involved depending especially upon the actual condition for which the medicine is given. Nor do we know the variable therapeutic effect dependent upon the doctor/patient interaction. Even if it ranged from only 0 to 10% then this economic model given would be relevant. Evidence put forward in this part of the book suggests, however, that the range may be anything from 0 to 50%.

At present, however, we lack an economic model that can quantify the health impact of the 'human effect'. A number of studies in this book have referred to effects such as reduced prescribing, less use of medical services, reduced hospital stay and other factors. Health planners of the future, however, will require firmer evidence than is available at present.

Summary

Three theories were proposed in this chapter to explain some of the work of the physician healer.

The first theory explored why and how a therapeutic encounter should lead to an improvement in the patient's condition. A number of processes are involved from patient expectation before the consultation to conditioned responses during and after the consultation. Other factors include an altered perceptual shift and changed behaviour following the consultation, which can lead to a cascade effect that amplifies the self-healing powers of the patient. Some of these processes are intrinsic to every consultation, while others depend upon on the patient, the doctor and the quality of the consultation.

The second theory examined the different types of role that a physician healer will need to adopt. Each of the roles – the provision of diagnosis and conventional treatment, of passive healing, of active healing and the role of director can be effective in its own place. The skilful physician healer will need to be proficient in each but also to adapt to whichever role is appropriate in a given circumstance. Clearly it will not be possible to make all patients more self-dependent, but nevertheless it is desirable to make an attempt in all. The pinnacle of success is when the patient becomes his/her own physician healer and the doctor is relegated to the sideline as advisor.

The third theory, based on health economics, explains why the physician healer is now coming to the fore as modern technology becomes increasingly unaffordable and frequently inappropriate in the context of many of the problems that present to us. The paradox is that as technology reaches its pinnacle, the therapeutic skills that preceded it have become evermore important – regardless of whether that technology is used. A report from the NHS Research and Development Health Technology Assessment Programme in 1999 concluded that an environment that fostered a strong patient/practitioner relationship was generally therapeutic and expressed concern at 'new cost conserving incentive structures (in the USA) that reduced the time that practitioners can personally spend with their patients to develop the type of relationship that will foster positive expectancies and maximise health gains'. Modern health economics suggests a new balance between the psychological, sociological, ecological aspects and the overemphasised technological sides of medical provision.

References

1 Horowitz RI, Horowitz SM (1993) Adherence to treatment and health outcomes. *Arch Intern Med*. **153**: 1863–8.

2 Spiegel D *et al.* (1989) Effect of psychosocial treatment on survival of patients with metastatic breast cancer. *Lancet*. **Oct 14**: 888–91.

3 Fawzy FI, Fawzy NW, Hyun CS *et al.* (1993) Malignant melanoma: effects of an early structured psychiatric intervention coping, and affective state on recurrence and survival 6 years later. *Arch Gen Psychiat*. **50**: 681.

4 Ratcliffe MA *et al.* (1995) Eysenck Personality Inventory L-scores in patients with Hodgkin's disease and Non-Hodgkin's lymphoma. *Psychooncology*. **4**: 39–45.

5 Fulder S (1996) *The Handbook of Complementary Medicine*. OUP, Oxford.

PART THREE

Theory into practice: how do we improve our effectiveness as physician healers?

Michael Dixon

Introduction

It is clear from previous chapters that the therapist and his/her 'non-specific healing skills' are frequently as important as the specific therapy that he/she gives. Indeed, it seems likely that variations in therapeutic outcome are often more a factor of variation in these skills than in purely clinical skills. One effect of the modern GP becoming highly skilled in modern medical techniques is that this may have led to a reduction in his/her ability to help patients combat complex disease processes, where modern medicine is less effective. Unfortunately, however, the focus is always on the doctor's clinical ability. Yet the importance of therapist over therapy has been suggested in a large number of studies. A review of the effectiveness of psychotherapy analysing 475 psychotherapy outcome studies concluded, for instance, that each therapeutic method had about equivalent effectiveness.[1] Previous studies that compared psychological, psychiatric and psychoanalytic approaches have also shown that the nature of the interaction between therapist and patient tends to be more important than the method used.

This section will try to use evidence, where it is available, but the aim is to be thought-provoking rather than didactic. As all GPs know, there is no fixed formula for a successful therapist and a GP that follows such a formula is likely to seem a fake. Technique and style have to be related to the personality of the GP and the patient – ultimately it is only the effect on the patient and not the excellence of the therapist that matters. GPs are by nature competitive and want to do their best, but seeking perfection as a therapist may be paradoxically quite damaging. The most perfect, knowledgeable and sensitive GP may (simply as a result of his/her omnipotence) serve to undermine the coping and self-healing powers of his/her patient. This is something that GPs frequently see in practice, when a spouse says that a recently departed partner was 'perfect'. This often implies a dependence that makes it difficult for the surviving spouse to pick up the threads of their life.

I remember one GP, when I entered practice, who was regarded as useless by many of his colleagues. Yet many patients were great fans of his and had developed self-healing skills and coping abilities simply because that they knew they had to! He was the catalyst that *they* needed to help them and they had recognised it. Thus, it is the signal that the patient receives that promotes the self-healing process. This is what matters and not the quality of the person sending the signal. This may be a difficult and confusing message for doctors who are used to the more clear cut messages of those who teach and assess them in their training.

Although the potential is always there (as we have seen in Part Two of this book) there are many consultations in which the successful GP healer may be unable to change a patient's symptoms or physical well-being. What he/she may do, however, is to change the patient's perception of him/herself, his/her presenting disease and his/her role in it. This may be involve a long learning process but an altered perception may end in the realisation that the patient him/herself is the essential factor in their health and well-being. The long-term effect may give the patient a better resistance to disease and these changes in one patient may have a healing effect on the society around him/her. Ryoichi Obitsu, a Japanese surgeon who combines complementary therapy with traditional surgical techniques in the treatment of cancer, puts it thus: 'The field of a patient, the field of a medical professional and the field of the family interact and influence each other and facilitate each other's growth. We must seek a structure of medical treatment that will make it possible to increase the harmony of one, then to influence each other'. The importance of the 'mind set' in this process cannot be underestimated but runs contrary to current medical teaching and research, which tends to emphasise short-term cause and effect.

It is this concentration on 'cause and effect that makes us think that the patient has come for 'something' and that it is up to us as doctors to produce the goods. Thus we are bound to see the patient in our own terms rather than those of the patient him/herself. Our actions may betray these projections and undermine the patient's self-healing powers by taking things over and actually depriving the patient of the very control that he or she needs so desperately. If there is one common theme in most consultations, it is that patients are hoping for some sort of control over the situation that they find themselves in. Much better that they find this control themselves but we should be prepared to do it for them when they cannot. In this context, we know from research that what they are looking for above anything is a message that they can understand, remember and use.

This whole area of 'messages' and 'mind sets' is at odds with the popular conception of a GP sitting poised with prescription pad and pen as the patient enters the room. The clinical training of the doctor and the prescription pad itself are important symbols and are frequently life-saving. As frequently, however, they are no more than symbols of a therapeutic encounter that has little to do with either.

Reference

1   Smith J *et al.* (1980) *The Benefits of Psychotherapy*. Johns Hopkins University Press, Baltimore.

CHAPTER TEN

Theory into practice I

The next three chapters will look at various aspects of our therapeutic role. They are in no particular order but the four categories in this chapter are aspects of every therapeutic encounter.

The doctor–patient relationship

We looked at evidence showing the therapeutic importance of the doctor–patient relationship in Chapter Four. It is possible for there to be a relationship between doctor and patient in only one encounter or for there to be an ongoing relationship as a result of many. Occasionally, perhaps we should stand back from the consultation and ask ourselves: 'Do I have a relationship with this patient? If so what kind of relationship? For whom? and Is it therapeutic?'

As we have seen, a large number of studies have confirmed that relationships are in themselves good for health.[1] Research on the specific relationship between doctor and patient confirmed that this is also therapeutically important as we saw at the end of Chapter Four. A positive relationship enables the patient to 'plug directly into the doctor'. Expectation theory predicts that the credibility of the therapist and the nature of the interpersonal relationship between patient and therapist will be crucial to the outcome of treatment. A number of studies have confirmed this and shown that the physician's attitude to the patient is regarded as very important by the patient him/herself.[2,3] We all like to be liked, respected and understood, and all the more so by someone whom we respect and like – especially when we are unwell. A relationship that works well will create its own feedback effects that will enhance both mood and relationship and allow the sort of cascade effects that were described in Chapter Nine. The importance of the therapeutic relationship explains why compliance with medication depends more upon the doctor than the personal characteristics of the patients.[4] In particular, a patient is much more likely to take a prescription if he thinks that he knows the prescribing doctor well.[5]

The basis of the relationship is trust and what a patient tells a doctor provides important feedback as to whether he or she regards the doctor as a safe haven for expressing feelings that really matter. From the patient's point of view a relationship becomes possible when he/she perceives that the doctor is concerned, the patient matters and the doctor is behind him/her.

A doctor that can make strong positive relationships with his/her patients is in a strong therapeutic position even before the medical encounter because the patient will already expect positive results. Past successes, big or small, tend to amplify such effects as every experienced GP knows. A dramatic visible success that is talked about locally can have profound effects on the therapeutic efficacy of a new doctor.

This being said – is it possible to provide a recipe for GPs wishing to increase their therapeutic potential by improving their doctor–patient relationships? One problem is that they are all so different that it is difficult to give a formula that will cover all possible relationships. Generalisations are possible, however, and certain traits in doctors are almost always helpful, for example approachability, adaptability, integrity, being able to deal with intimacy and being non-judgmental. Mutual respect, trust and liking are also important aspects of most positive relationships.

Increasing emphasis on personal lists and continuity of care have encouraged the development of such positive relationships. Conditioned by past kindness and positive consultations, the relationship should provide a healing effect both in making the patient feel more secure generally and prior to making a consultation when he/she is ill. A familiar face in times of danger is always welcome. At worst the patient may say of this relationship – 'Better the devil you know than the devil you don't'. The implication is that sometimes it is the fact of a relationship that counts rather than the specific or non-specific therapeutic skills of the doctor!

The importance of offering continuity is evidenced by a number of studies. It seems that if we can offer some degree of continuity of care then our patients will be more satisfied with their care.[6] They are also more likely to take their medications correctly and have their problems identified by their physician.[7] Conversely, if we fail to offer continuity then it seems that this is associated with additional morbidity in our patients and a tendency to see the GP more often and also to cancel appointments more frequently.[8] Continuity of care is also important in reducing the need for hospital admission and is thus an important factor in a cost-effective health service.[9,10]

Getting the relationship right is thus not only important if we are to make our patients better, but also an important means of saving money for technological medicine where it is needed and more appropriate. The doctor who can provide therapeutic relationships in the surgery and catalyse therapeutic relationships outside in the locality is thus providing a service that has a direct impact both on health and the health economy.

The nature of the therapeutic relationship and how we can develop it is currently an ongoing topic of research at the Institute of General Practice at Exeter University – hopefully it will not be long before it can be described more fully than has been possible here.

Therapeutic authority

Most patients need to feel that their doctor is therapeutically effective. The need to believe that he/she can take on his/her arbitrary and feared symptoms and subject them to some sort of control. This need to believe in your doctor is witnessed by exclamations such as 'of course he saved my uncle's life' or 'he's one of the top ones'. Therapeutic authority can come with a medical degree especially if the doctor is a 'professor' or 'specialist'. It can also be gained by reputation and past successes. Factors such as age, experience or recent medical training will be viewed as positive or negative according to the patient's perspective.

A patient's attitudes to his/her own doctor's therapeutic skills will be derived from his views on medicine in general and opinions from those around him, but also from his own perceived experiences with that particular doctor. Previous experiences, for instance, when the doctor has sutured a wound, delivered a baby or attended a child, will all be taken into account even before the patient enters the consulting room.

The point here is that it is not the *actual skills* of the doctor that matter in this context but his skills as perceived by the patient. That is what counts even though, as we all know, patients can get it very wrong! Of course, this begs the question of whether they have actually got it wrong if they actually get better. Having human skills is no excuse for a doctor losing his/her clinical skills, but the former may be more important in many circumstances.

Consequently, a doctor should be concerned about his/her reputation as a bad reputation will damage the therapeutic encounter. Conversely, a supportive partnership within a given general practice will emphasise the positive aspects of all health professionals involved as well as the specialists that are referred to by the practice. Each will bathe in a reflected light, which eventually shines on the patient, whose own judgement is validated.

So where does a 'good reputation' come from? A bit of luck helps, but perceived expertise may be as much a factor of the skills outlined in this and future chapters as the skilled application of evidence-based clinical pathways. The patients are bound to vary in the ways that they make their judgements. In left-brain-dominant patients extensive discussion may be necessary before a patient perceives the doctor as having therapeutic authority, while less cognitive patients may be put off by a doctor that talks too much.[11] Listen to the patient and he/she will tell you what he/she understands as the criteria of a competent doctor.

Magic/mystery

If a therapeutic process is beyond a patient's comprehension, there is a tendency in some to lend it a degree of credibility that is out of all proportion to its actual effectiveness. This credibility may greatly amplify its effectiveness. This may be frequently the case in orthodox medicine, where the doctor 'speaks in tongues' because he overestimates the level of comprehension of his/her patient and conveys an impression that his medicine is a learned, complex and a somewhat magical process. Many patients are also attracted by the magical nature of alternative therapies, which often seem more exotic and aesthetic than conventional medical treatment.

The ECG machine, the Doppler machine and even the stethoscope may also seem 'magical' to patients. The distinction between diagnostics and therapeutics may be lost on the very young and the very old, who may in some vague way see tapping reflexes or X-rays as therapeutic. The effect, of course, is much greater with specialist care, which has many more powerful effects such as lasers and computer scans. A similar magic was practised by some of the old fashioned healers. For instance, Zouave Jacob, a nineteenth century French healer, would have no truck with concepts such as empathy or positive relationships. He was described as 'disagreeable, awkward and inclined to stamp with such a rude violence on the floor that the casement shook'. Nevertheless 'when he passed along a row of low wooden benches lined with sick and crippled people who could not walk, everyone would rise and stand erect'.

Most doctors would think it inappropriate to encourage their patients' magical fantasies about modern medical science but receiving therapy in a consultation will always be different from buying it over the counter. As doctors, we may notice this least of all. The magical effect of unfamiliar therapies can be explained to some extent by conditioning theory, which would predict that where there is 'placebo sag' to one particular mode (such as tablets bought over the counter) then placebo effectiveness will be restored by changing to a different mode (e.g. consulting a doctor). The magic/mystery effect of some alternative therapies may be explained by the new and strange environment being a catalyst that allows the patient to view himself differently and thereby change and redirect the forces that kept him unwell.

Thus a patient's preconceptions as to the 'magical' nature of medicine and its therapies will have a bearing upon his hopefulness as he approaches the consultation. They will also have a bearing on the effectiveness of that consultation. Most doctors do not like consciously using magic but they need to be aware of its effect on their patients. If a patient needs magic it may be cruel to deny it. A patient may want to be understood but equally he/she may want an image of the doctor, which is different from the person that he sits next to in the pub. Too much informality may thus in some patients have a negative therapeutic effect but this should not imply that remoteness is a good thing either.

The 'magician' doctor has to be different things at different times. A therapeutically credible 'fat controller' of the patient's welfare and purveyor of magic on some occasions. Understanding, approachable, equal and facilitating the patient's self-healing powers on others. Frequently the GP may need to be both in the same consultation. Testimony to the fact that we are dealing with real people frequently in a heightened emotional state. This is territory where logic and concepts such as 'doing the right thing' go out the window. Intuition and timing are everything and have been undervalued in the modern general practice consultation.

Time/attention

It may seem odd to put forward the concept that giving time and attention is a therapeutic technique. Especially, when every GP knows that this is the thing that we lack most of all. Professor Denis Pereira Gray, however, has pointed out that we may have more time than we think. The average patient is seen for 9.4 minutes and consults five times a year, which means that we see him altogether for 47 minutes a year. Furthermore, the average patient is registered for 11 years and during this time we would therefore see him/her for an average of 8½ hours! Many of those patients, where the therapeutic effect is particularly important, will have been seen for even longer.

The benefits of simply giving time and attention have been demonstrated in studies ranging from the treatment of dental fear using a placebo control group, to the treatment of schizophrenics.[12,13] Varying amounts of time are required to understand the patient's problem and his/her worries concerning it.

Furthermore, we should not underestimate the value of our simply being available and 'just being there', especially given the important healing effect of our perceived role as doctors. Doctors see listening as important in the diagnostic process but possibly underrate its therapeutic value. Research in general practice shows that in shorter consultations (five as opposed to ten minutes) fewer problems are identified and patients are less satisfied with the consultation.[14] Patients given shorter consultations are more likely to return within four weeks with a new illness episode and will tend to have a higher consultation rate.[15] Less preventative care is given in shorter consultations and there seems to be an inverse relationship between consultation length and a tendency to prescribe.[16]

Some doctors seem to be able to give their patients the illusion they have all the time in the world, while others, given the same amount of time, seem hurried and dismissive to their patients. Time, as we have said, is the scarcest of all commodities in general practice. Patients know that, which is precisely why they value so highly any GP who is prepared to give it. Paradoxically, some highly skilled physicians will feel that it is a waste of their time to sit around listening, when they should be getting on with practising their more technical skills.

Being hassled and short of time is a genuine phenomenon in modern general practice and can sometimes be put to therapeutic effect in terms of encouraging a patient to be more self-dependent. It should not be used, however, as a means of raising the perceived status of the doctor and demeaning the comparative importance and self-esteem of the patient.

Summary

Central to the effectiveness of the physician healer is the relationship that he/she has with the patients. Relationships can be destructive and indulgent, but conversely they can be central to the therapy. Analysing why a relationship is poor and how to improve it may be the key to therapeutic success. Clinical competence is important but a patient's 'fantasies' of the clinical competence of his/her doctor are equally important.

Establishing therapeutic authority depends partly upon reputation and past success but colleagues have a role. Part of our therapeutic authority comes from our role as 'guardians of medical magic'. We can use our magic wisely and amplify the effects of our therapeutic techniques. Conversely, as magicians we need to be aware that we are playing with fire and should not use this magic to disable our patients. Finally, we must sometimes put our problem-solving and goal-orientated selves to one side and recognise that simply 'being there' can sometimes be the most important treatment of all. It is not only therapeutic in itself but when 'the great man/woman' spares a few extra minutes for the patient, this conveys strong messages about the patient's own importance and worth. 'He/she gives me time' is a frequent and positive comment made by patients of their doctors, and probably reflects their actual needs.

References

1 Berkman LF (1995) The role of social relations in health promotion. *Psychosom Med.* **57**: 245–54.

2 DiMatteo MR, DiNicola DD (1982) Social science and the art of medicine: from Hippocrates to holism. In: HS Friedman, MR DiMatteo (eds) *Interpersonal Issues in Healthcare*. Academic Press, New York.

3 Wickramasekera IA (1985) A conditioned response model of the placebo effect: predictions from the model. In: L White, T Tursky, GE Schwartz (eds) *Placebo: theory, research and mechanisms*. The Guilford Press, New York.

4 Evans L, Spelman M (1983) The problem of non-compliance with drug therapy. *Drugs* **25** (1): 63–76.

5 Ettlinger PR, Freeman GK (1981) General practice compliance study: is it worth being a personal doctor? *BMJ – Clin Res.* **282** (6271): 1192–4.

6 Wasson JH, Sauvigne AE, Mogielnicki RP *et al.* (1984) Continuity of outpatient medical care in elderly men: a randomised trial. *JAMA.* **252**: 2413–17.

7 Becker MH, Drachman RH, Kirscht JP (1974) Continuity of

pediatrician: new support for an old shibboleth. *J Pediatr*. **84**: 599–605.

8   Sweeney K, Pereira Gray DJ (1995) Patients who do not receive continuity of care from their general practitioner. *Br J Gen Pract*. **4**: 153–8.

9   Weiss LJ, Blustein J (1996) Faithful patients: the effect of long term physician–patient relationships on the costs and use of healthcare by older Americans. *Am J Public Health*. **86**: 1742–7.

10   James M, Gill MD, Mainous G (1998) The role of provider continuity in preventing hospitalisations. *Arch Fam Med*. **7**: 352–7.

11   Cacioppo JT, Petty RE (1982) The need for cognition. *J Pers Soc Psychol*. **42**: 116–31.

12   Bernstein DA, Klein K (1982) Multiple approach to dental fear. *J Behav Ther Exp Psychiat*. **13**: 289–92.

13   Meurice E (1986) Overall results of attempts to trear schizophrenia by hemodialysis. Reflections on the placebo effect in a psychosis. *(French) Acta Psychiat Belg*. **86** (3): 266–86.

14   Morrell DC, Evans ME, Morris RW, Roland MO (1986) The 'five minute' consultation: effect of time constraint on clinical content and patient satisfaction. *BMJ – Clin Res*. **292** (6524): 870–3.

15   Hughes D (1983) Consultation length and outcome in two group general practices. *J R Coll Gen Practitioners*. **33**: 143–7.

16   Murray TS, Borber JH, Hanway DR (1978) Consulting time and prescribing rates. *Update*. **16**: 969–75.

CHAPTER ELEVEN

Theory into practice II

Chapter Ten described several aspects that are an inevitable part of the consultation. In this chapter we look at therapeutic effects, which are not necessarily part of every consultation. No doctor will be hauled to a medical hearing for failing to provide them but few can be therapeutically effective if they fail to offer any of them.

Empathy

Empathy, kindness, comfort and understanding would all seem to be intuitively therapeutic – benefiting both the patient's emotional state and the doctor–patient relationship. The need to provide such things can, however, seem an unwanted interruption to the thoughts of the modern medical practitioner as he/she pursues the intellectual processes of the diagnosis and treatment. All the more so when the need to provide comfort and empathy is often a reflection of his/her inability to provide 'effective' treatment for the problem in hand. Furthermore, it is tiring to dispense kindness and empathy all day. Not surprisingly then, the task is often partially delegated to others.

Yet empathy is an important part of the therapeutic process. If the doctor appears to understand the patient's problem then the patient is more likely to perceive an improvement.[1] Patients with chronic illnesses improve better with consultations in which they are able to follow their own (rather than the doctor's) agenda and in which they are able to express their emotions.[2] Lack of warmth in parental relations has been shown to lead to a higher likelihood of the later development of cancer.[3] Good supportive relationships, however, have been shown to have a large number of beneficial consequences varying from the prevention of heart attacks to a reduction in serum cholesterol and uric acid.[4,5] Intimacy in relationships has also been related to better physical and mental health.[6]

Is empathy something that we are born with or that we can develop? Warmth and a positive emotional attitude, as well as simply spending time with the patient, has been shown to be a major factor in whether the patient feels cared for.[7] Empathy is, however, a reciprocal arrangement between patient and doctor, which is why it amplifies the health and well-being of the patient. EEG studies on patients seeing healers suggest that there is frequently a synchronisation of EEG patterns suggesting that empathy might be measurable. Whether on an electro-physiological level or an emotional one, synchronicity is clearly a vital component in empathy. Getting it right in the consultation is not about being slushy and nice but requires a deep intelligence far removed from simply following a treatment protocol. It is, therefore, not surprising to find that excellence in empathic accuracy is far more likely in those who are especially intelligent and cognitively complex.[8]

Rogers[9] described how the triad of empathy, warmth and genuineness provide the necessary and sufficient conditions for change in a patient. So we should not be surprised that having failed to provide anything 'useful' during a consultation, the patient often says to us on leaving something along the lines of 'Thank you for listening' or 'Thank you for being so understanding'. 'Caritas', it now seems in the light of modern research, is as much about curing as it is about caring.

Relaxation

We have already seen in Part Two of this book that unrelieved stress has harmful medical effects in both animals and humans. Conversely, interventions that increase a feeling of calmness can improve immune function and increase energy.[10] We have also seen how relaxation treatment can improve survival time for cancer patients (e.g. with breast cancer, melanoma and non-Hodgkin's lymphoma).

We know that couples with poor relationships tend to stress each other physiologically when they meet.[11] Similarly a poor relationship between therapist and patient may lead to harmful physiological effects, while a good relationship should improve things. Complementary therapists are particularly skilful at putting patients in a relaxed state during the consultation. As patients feel better in this way, they then notice their negative symptoms less. This is the case with pain, for instance, which is perceived as worse if the patient is stressed, depressed or fearful. Furthermore, in the relaxed state, patients are better able to take on information that is informative, reassuring and positive.

As doctors, we should perhaps attempt to get our patients into a relaxed state from the moment they enter the waiting room. The reception area of a surgery is thus a first stage in the patient's treatment. Is it uplifting to the spirit or is it just medically correct? We have already seen the importance of the environment and therapeutic setting and problems such as lost notes or frequent telephone calls are likely to affect the degree to which a patient can relax in the surgery.[12] Most important of all, however, will be the skilfulness of the doctor in putting the patient at his/her ease and this may depend to some extent upon the state of mind of the doctor.

Reassurance

Doctors are much better placed to give reassurance with their detailed technical knowledge than any other therapist. The sort of relationship they have with their patients and their own therapeutic authority should be major contributors to their effectiveness in giving such reassurance.

Balint condemned the misuse of reassurance by GPs, when it was blind reassurance without a satisfactory diagnosis having been made. Appropriate reassurance is, however, an important part of the physician/healer role. Where there is straightforward physical disease (and especially where there is not) reassurance about its nature, pattern and prognosis may be very therapeutic. Where precise reassurance is not possible, a patient may need a different sort of reassurance. For instance, he/she may be comforted in knowing that his/her symptoms fit a pattern or he/she may need reassurance about him/herself (e.g. that he/she is not going mad) or about him/herself in relation to others (e.g. that it is a common problem). A patient recently reported: 'A lady gynaecologist told me that most ladies leak a little – it was very reassuring and I am not so worried about it any more'.

Another example in point was made recently to one of the authors by a patient commenting on a consultation with her doctor: 'He said that he didn't know what I had and that he wasn't going to give me anything but that I would get better – which I did!' Reassurance in this sense may be as therapeutic as providing an exact diagnosis or prescription. This was suggested by a study on 200 patients who were either given a diagnosis and medication or told that there was no evidence of disease and they required no treatment.[13] The therapeutic effectiveness of both approaches was the same. Furthermore, a reassured patient will be less anxious and is more likely to comply with any medication that is given.[14]

If reassurance can show that the doctor, or better still the patient, has some control over the situation, then this must have a positive healing effect. We have already seen this in the animal and human studies mentioned in Part Two of this book, which showed that the process of restoring control led to improvements in the neuroendocrine-immunological axis. One reaction to perceived illness may be for the patient to see a disease or injured part as separate from him/herself and one effect of reassurance may be to restore a sense of harmony.

Touch

Many complementary therapies involve a lot of touching. Touch is almost always emotionally significant. Being touched is, for most, a pleasant experience in itself and carries the implication of feeling accepted. The old, the unloved and the chronically sick have been described by Bernie Siegel, as being 'skin starved'. As one patient put it to the author recently: 'I've got no one to hug me'. Touch is particularly important for these patients. Many of them may be in need of urgent 'body psychotherapy'.

This may explain why massage for their musculoskeletal pains often seems to be more effective than evidence-based medical remedies. Yet we relentlessly push a whole host of medications at them in order to try and cure their ailments and unhappiness. Those kitchen cupboards full of unused pills are testimony that we got it wrong – the patient wanted caring not medicines.

All of us have been conditioned since our childhood to get better with touch ever since our mother put her arm round us and kissed us when we were unwell or had accidents. Whether or not touch involves some other therapeutic process is unknown. Hippocrates, writing around the turn of the fifth century, said 'it is believed by experienced doctors that the heat which oozes out of the hand, when being applied to the sick, is highly salutary – it has often appeared, while I have been soothing my patients, as if there was a singular property in my hands to pull and draw away from the affected parts, aches and diverse impurities, by laying my hand upon the place, and by extending my fingers towards it'.[15] The Japanese surgeon Ryoichi Obitsu puts it slightly differently: 'I have my field of life and the patient has his/her field of life, and both are connected though breath and skin. There is a shared field between us. The concept is that two people try to restore the order in the shared field'. This view would see physical proximity as a therapeutic quantity independent of actual touch.

In every consultation there is incidental touching (e.g. during an examination), social touching and what healers have described as 'therapeutic touching'. Some doctors will probably provide therapeutic touch as described by Hippocrates and be unaware of it. It is, however, a method that can also be learnt.[16] Experienced physicians often consciously take a patient's pulse (as an examination touch) as a means of communicating warmth and extending hospitality (e.g. social touch). Where the significance of such touch is unconscious for both physician and patient it is likely that there will be a therapeutic effect as a result of the unconscious associations in the mind of the patient. Thus, at whatever level the doctor touches his patients, from the incidental to the explicitly therapeutic, there is likely to be some healing effect.

Improving the patient's self-esteem

Many of our chronically ill patients are demoralised and have poor self-esteem. This may be a primary or secondary factor in their illness. A patient with poor self-esteem feels that he/she is not worth curing and furthermore assumes that he/she does not have the strength to help him/herself. Thus the patient with poor self-esteem renounces autonomy and is not surprised that he/she can be helped by nobody.

It is tempting, using the medical model to see our patients as their normal selves plus their presenting symptoms. If this was so then experimental studies on pain in normal subjects (with a placebo effect of 9–16%) would show similar results to patients actually complaining of pain (with a placebo effect of 30–40%). It seems that our symptoms actually change us in all sorts of subtle ways affecting our self-confidence and our ability to get better. This is why the physician healer is so effective with patients who are genuinely ill. It may be why his/her skills are underestimated by health planners and commentators, who are not.

Conversely, therefore, improving a patient's self-esteem should make his/her symptoms and problems seem less bad and make him/her feel that he/she is both able to be cured and worth curing. How can we do this?

The therapist may improve the patient's self-esteem directly by giving him/her messages that he/she is special, important, unique and able. This may be particularly effective in the English culture where, unlike the American culture, such messages tend to be underplayed. Equally, the patient may get these messages indirectly and perhaps more subtly as a function of the way in which the therapist behaves towards him/her. He/she may see that the doctor bothers, which suggests that the patient matters and we have already see how therapeutically powerful such messages can be in Part Two of this book. As a result of seeing that the doctor cares about him/her the patient's self-esteem improves and also with it his/her faith in him/herself and his/her healing resources. Complementary therapists are particularly skilled at both sorts of process.

Nevertheless, in conventional medical treatment we often do

exactly the opposite. We may inadvertently lower the patient's self-esteem by taking treatment out of their hands and ignoring their own role in their treatment. We may also belittle them when we are trying to reassure them when we make comments such as: 'I can't find anything wrong with you', 'It's nothing to worry about', 'I expect its just due to stress'.

For many patients therefore, it may be necessary for them to feel good about themselves in the first place before they can feel positive towards their treatment and outcome. Furthermore, any physician that successfully improves a patient's self-esteem will also improve his/her general sense of well-being and this may itself be an important and independent outcome of the therapeutic encounter.

Treating the individual

Conditioning theory has shown us how each person's healing response is very much related to a long line of previous experience stretching back into childhood. Thus, a doctor who takes into account a patient's beliefs, past experiences and expectation is far more likely to be successful than one who does not. Such individual attention will also tell the patient that the therapist cares about him and will improve not only his own self-esteem, but also his attitude towards the competence of the therapist. Some doctors are intolerant of the idiosyncratic beliefs of their patients, especially when they have no 'scientific validity'. Expectancy theory tells us that we should go along with these beliefs, especially if we are unable to change them, as confrontation between patient and doctor is unlikely to be therapeutic. If a patient tells a doctor (as one did recently) 'I don't believe in antibiotics', she is not only telling you what she believes but also about what will or will not be therapeutic for her. Thus we need to explore the patient's ideas and expectations and tailor advice and instructions to the details that we know about a patient's life.[17]

This is more difficult, of course, if the doctor does not know the patient very well. An elderly lady patient recently described an encounter with a locum doctor following a bout of gastroenteritis:

'I wasn't smitten by him. He told me that I could go out and eat a curry but I have never eaten curry in my life. He said it was due to a bug but when I asked him where the bug had come from, he said that it just came through the window'. The lady concerned was inferring subtly that the doctor had insufficiently recognised either herself or her medical problem. The result was an unnecessary second visit by her regular doctor the following day.

Complementary therapies tend to offer a very patient-orientated system of treatment. Medical treatments, however, tend to be disease orientated and therefore relatively impersonal. The patient may view him/herself as on a conveyor belt and some outpatient clinics may seem more like cattle markets than treatment centres. GPs are personal doctors and should therefore be in the business of offering personal medicine.[18] Their treatment should thus lie somewhere between the extreme individualism of some complementary therapies and the impersonality of some standard medical treatments. Doctors with an interest in personal medicine have developed the art of directing their full attention to the patient him/herself and tailoring therapy to their individual needs.

Modern research in general practice has supported the view that a patient-centred (as opposed to a disease-centred) approach, is healing. Patient-centred consultations have been associated with patients feeling understood and resolution of both their concerns and their symptoms.[19] Conversely, disease-centred consultations tend to result in the prescription of symptomatic medication and be shorter.[20] The degree to which the GP treats the 'whole patient' is related to the likelihood that the patient will take his/her medication, as well as the health outcome.[21]

So how does one treat the patient as an individual? Smiling, nodding and speaking warmly are related to the likelihood that a patient will tell you what is really wrong.[22] Eye contact is important and it is a means of showing the patient that he/she has the physician's full attention.[23] Allowed to tell his/her fully story, the patient needs to know that the physician has fully understood it and patients will vary as to whether they want simply reflective feedback or self-enhancing information.[24] Inevitably, the highly individualised consultation will have the effect of improving a patient's self-esteem with all the attendant benefits described above. Nevertheless, the patient-centred consultation, while being more rewarding and effective, can also be more stressful because the physician has to give more. Allowing the doctor a longer consultation time may be a necessary part of reducing such stress.[25]

Laughter

A recently bereaved patient was telling one of the authors about her late husband. She was describing her sadness and how much she was missing him. The author wanting to comfort her and having nothing better to say made the remark: 'Although he's dead, I am sure that he is still listening to you'. The patient creased up in laughter with the remark 'Well that would surprise me – he never did when he was alive!'

Laughter improves the emotional state and being able to laugh gives the message that doctor and patient can control and get above the situation. It is also an important means of bonding between patient and therapist. It tells each that they have a common view on life, which reflects their common humanity. In physiological terms, laughter is also followed by the relaxation response with all the attendant benefits that have already been discussed.

Suggestion/inspiration

The attitude of the physician and his enthusiasm for any given treatment have been shown to have dramatic effects on the outcome of treatment.[26-28] A doctor who is enthusiastic about his/her treatment will also ensure better compliance.

Not surprisingly then, patients with positive expectations do better. For instance, patients with chronic bronchitis have been shown to have greater exercise tolerance if they believe their treatment to be efficacious.[29] This also explains the positive influence of branded drugs.[30] The effect is seen even when the medication is ineffective, as was shown in one trial showing reduction of symptoms in healing of ulcers in patients given a treatment that was found to be therapeutically inactive.[31] Finally, the effect is also present when no medication is given as was demonstrated in one trial for patients with depression.[32]

Thomas[33] has shown that a positive consultation will lead to a greater improvement in symptoms than a negative consultation. Indeed the nature of the consultation (i.e. positive or negative) is a more important determinant of outcome than whether treatment is given.

Doctors do not like to see themselves as salesmen and many think that it is unethical to knowingly give a patient a placebo. This should not stop them reinforcing, however, the beneficial effects of any treatment that they believe to be effective. That is to say 'enhancing the expectation effect'. Conversely, they should be aware that if they give negative messages then this is likely to have a detrimental effect on outcome.[34] Guidance on the good effects that are to be expected (and possibly even side-effects) will encourage the patient to perceive these effects and will further amplify any improvement when it occurs.

We have already seen that suggestion can be effective in patients with tonsillitis and those with post-appendicectomy pain.[35,36] Effective suggestion emphasises the positive aspects of the situation and treatment and the messages need to be specific, in simple language and repeated sufficiently often enough for the patient to remember them. The more relaxed the patient is, the more likely is the suggestion to be taken in, remembered, stored and ultimately effective.

Not surprisingly, from all that has been said, any suggestions need to fit within the individual and cultural environment of the patient. A patient of the author recently gave a vivid example of how he had been recommended an 'unbeatable' (in fact quite ordinary) analgesic by a friend. The friend had told him: 'It's what they give the Coldstream Guards'. Not surprisingly the remedy had worked! Suggestion is a powerful instrument that can be misused. The opposite, that is to under-sell and render ineffective treatment that can have beneficial consequences to the patient, is a neglect of the doctor's therapeutic potential.

Hope

Everyone needs hope. It is also therapeutic. Whether naturally occurring or catalysed by the doctor, hope has been shown to alter outcome in patients wanting to lose weight. Optimism is also helpful to the outcome of patients with heart disease.[37]

What about the situation where there is no hope? Our expectations frequently become less realistic as things get worse. Hope is a variable entity that might range from the hope of a cure to the hope that a patient might live until the end of the week. Conventional wisdom dictates that patients are given realistic assessments of their situation. Few, however, can live without hope. It is, therefore, appropriate to also give an optimistic assessment within the bounds of realism so that the patient has something better to aim at. The further they aim, the further they get.

Nothing can be more cruel than to deny hope to a patient that needs it. TS Elliot put it better: 'Human kind cannot bear very much reality'.

Summary

Modern research has shown that empathy and caring are not simply a courtesy in the medical encounter. They are also important elements in enabling a patient to overcome and withstand illness. Treatment is also more likely to succeed when the doctor can provide proper reassurance, preferably in a relaxed atmosphere. Physical touch and physical presence are in themselves important therapeutic effects, especially in those who are least exposed to them on a daily basis. Patients are not simply a collection of illnesses and symptoms. Therapy will often be more successful if the physician is supportive and can boost the patient's self-confidence, and treat him/her as an individual rather than as part of a conveyor belt.

Humour provides an important means of vanquishing despair and escaping the vulnerability of disease. Suggestion is an important means of amplifying the effect of any given treatment, while hope is something few of us can do without altogether.

References

1   Stewart MA, McWhinney IR, Buck CW (1979) The doctor–patient relationship and its effect upon outcome. *J R Coll Gen Practitioners*. **29**: 77–82.

2   Kaplin SH, Greenfields S, Ware JE (1989) Assessing the effects of physician–patient interactions on the outcomes of chronic disease. *Med Care*. **27** (3): S110–S27.

3   Thomas CB, Duszynski KR, Shaffer JW (1979) Family attitudes reported in youth as potential predictors of cancer. *Psychosom Med*. **41**: 287–302.

4   Medalie JH *et al.* (1973) 5 year myocardial infarct incidence. *J Chron Dis*. **26**: 329–49.

5   Cobbs J (1974) Physiologic changes in men whose jobs were abolished. *J Psychosom Res*. **18**: 245–58.

6   Reis HT (1984) Social interaction and well-being. In: SW Duck (ed) *Personal Relationships: repairing personal relationships*, vol 5. Academic Press, London.

7   Elliott R, James E (1989) Varieties of client experience in psychotherapy: an analysis of the literature. *Clin Psychol Rev*. **9**: 443–67.

8   Davis MH, Kraus LA ((1997) Personality and empathic accuracy. In: W Ickes (ed.) *Empathic Accuracy*. Guilford Press, New York.

9   Rogers CR (1957) The necessary and sufficient conditions of therapeutic personality change. *J Consult Psychol*. **21**: 95–103.

10 Gruzelier J, Smith F, Nagy A *et al.* (2000) Prophylactic benefits at exam time on cell medicated immunity through self hypnosis training. Submitted for publication.

11 Burman B, Margolin G (1992) Analysis of the association between martial relationships and health problems: an interactional perspective. *Psychol Bull*. 1992: **112**: 39–63.

12 Ulrich R (1984) View through a window may influence recovery from surgery. *Science*. **224**: 420–1.

13 Thomas KB (1978) The consultation and the therapeutic illusion. *BMJ.* **1** (6123): 1327–8.

14 Evans L, Spelman M (1983) The problem of non-compliance with drug therapy. *Drugs.* **25** (1): 63–76.

15 Harvey D (1983) *The Power to Heal.* Aquarian Press, London.

16 Regan G, Shapiro D (1988) *The Healer's Handbook.* Element Books, Shaftesbury.

17 Tuckett D, Boulton M, Olsen C *et al.* (1985) *Meetings Between Experts: an approach to sharing ideas in medical consultations.* Tavistock Publications, London.

18 Pereira Gray DJ (1978) Feeling at home. *J R Coll Gen Practitioners.* **28**: 6–17.

19 Fehrsen GS, Henbest RJ (1993) In search of excellence. Expanding the patient-centred clinical method: a three stage assessment. Department of Family Medicine, Medunsa, Republic of South Africa. *Fam Pract.* **10** (1): 49–54.

20 Department of General Practice, University of Edinburgh (1992) Attitudes to medical care, the organisation of work, and stress among general practitioners. *Br J Gen Pract.* **42** (358): 181–5.

21 Safran DG, Taira DA, Rogers WH *et al.* (1998) Linking primary care performance to outcomes of care. *J Fam Pract.* **47**: 213–20.

22 Pope B, Siegman A (1968) Interviewer warmth in relation to interviewee verbal behaviour. *J Consult Clin Psychol.* **32**: 588–95.

23 Ellsworth PC, Calsmith JM (1973) Eye contact and gaze aversion in aggressive encounters. *J Person Soc Psychol.* **33**: 117–33.

24 Sedikides C (1993) Assessment, enhancement and verification determinants of the self-evaluation process. *J Person Soc Psychol.* **65**: 317-338.

25 Henbest RJ, Fehrsen GS (1992) Patient-centredness: is it applicable outside the west? Its measurement and effect on outcomes. Department of Family Medicine, Medical University of Southern Africa, Medunsa. *Fam Pract.* **9** (3): 311–17.

26 Hahan RA (1985) A sociolocultural model of illness and healing. In: L White, B Tursky, GE Schwartz. *Placebo: theory, research and mechanisms.* The Guilford Press, New York.

27 Benson H, Epstein MD (1975) The placebo effect: a neglected asset in the care of patients. *JAMA.* **232** (12): 1225.

28 DiMatteo MR, DiNicola DD (1982) *Achieving Patient*

Compliance: the psychology of the medical practitioner's role. Pergamon Press, New York.

29 Morgan AD, Peck EF, Buchanan DR, McHardy GJR (1983) Effects of attitudes and beliefs on exercise tolerance in chronic bronchitis. *BMJ.* **296**: 171–3.

30 Branthwaite A, Cooper P (1981) Analgesic effects of branding in treatment of headaches. *BMJ.* **282**: 1576–8.

31 MacDonald AJ, Peden NR, Hayton R *et al.* (1980) Symptoms relief and the placebo effect in the trial of an anti-pectic drug. *Gut.* **21**: 323–6.

32 Rabkin JG, McGrath PJ, Quitkin FM *et al.* (1990) Effects of pill-giving on maintenance of placebo response in patients with chronic mild depression. *Am J Psychiat.* **147**: 1622–6.

33 Thomas KB (1987) General practice consultations: is there any point in being positive? *BMJ – Clin Res.* **294** (6581): 1200–2.

34 Daniels AM, Sallie R (1981) Headache, lumbar puncture and expectation. *Lancet* **i**: 1003.

35 Olsson B, Olsson B, Tibblin G (1989) Effect of patients' expectations on recovery from acute tonsillitis. *Fam Pract.* **6** (3): 188–92.

36 Egbert LD, Battit GE, Welch CE, Bartlett MK (1964) Reduction of postoperative pain by encouragement and instruction of patients. *NEJM.* **270**: 825–7.

37 Scheier MF, Matthews KA, Owens JF *et al.* (1989) Dispositional optimism and recovery from coronary artery by-pass surgery: the beneficial effects on psychological wellbeing. *J Person Soc Psychol.* **57:** 1024–10.

CHAPTER TWELVE

Theory into practice III

In this chapter we begin to explore some of the ways in which a patient can actively help him/herself and develop self-healing capabilities. It is crucially dependent upon the doctor enabling the patient to take a more positive approach and role in health and illness. As passive turns to active, losers turn to winners and the locus of control moves from doctor to patient. As the patient becomes more actively involved in his/her treatment, he/she will seek out those things which may be of benefit. As an agent of change rather than a victim of problems, the patient sees his/her own central role in promoting good health. The doctor and his/her medication become, in many respects, ancillary.

One obvious benefit of patients achieving this active role is that it is bound to save scarce doctors' time and resources. Doctors who are able to change the 'scripts' of patients in this way are also performing a vital public health role as this will not only effect the health of that individual patient, but also that of his/her family and all those around.

There is also much evidence that this frame of mind has important clinical benefits. We have already seen how active coping behaviour can improve survival in breast cancer, malignant melanoma and Hodgkin's disease, as well as preventing the recurrence of genital herpes. A recent paper on chronic fatigue syndrome concluded that a good prognosis depended mostly on a positive illness attitude and coping style.[1] Research reported so far in psychoneuroimmunology suggests that the patient in an active state will be much more resistant to disease. Indeed compliance studies show that simply taking a treatment (which infers a positive attitude to it) reduces the risk of death by one-third regardless of what treatment one is taking.[2] Quite apart from being able to improve current disease, a positive frame of mind is also likely to make a patient more resistant to harmful behaviours and future disease.

These points can be illustrated by looking at the main killer disease in the UK. Most doctors and patients would accept that coronary artery disease can be largely prevented by changes in behaviour and attitude. It does, however, come as something of a surprise to find that even established coronary artery disease can be reversed by behavioural change.[3] A study involving changes in diet, exercise and stress management resulted in dramatic changes that were similar to those seen with cholesterol-lowering drugs and also resulted in the reversal of established coronary artery stenosis as measured by coronary ateriography. Most surprisingly, such changes were most marked in those patients who had the most severe coronary artery disease, and the improvement in pain severity ($p = .0006$) and the diameter of the stenosis ($p = .001$) all occurred within only one year. Why is clinical medicine failing to shout such messages loud and clear? It appears that we are so dazzled by specialist procedures and modern drugs that we can no longer believe that it is possible to achieve such impressive results without them or to vastly improve the effects of such drugs and procedures when the mind and orthodox medical treatment are working in parallel.

How can we help patients to get into the active mode?

This is probably the most important question in medicine. It is also probably the greatest challenge to the doctor/healer especially when faced with the non-compliant, the dependent, the 'yes but' and the despondent. It requires a doctor with inspiration, flare, motivation, understanding and determination. In some ways a bulldozer, who will accept that no case is hopeless and that the classical 'heart sinks' are simply a challenge. A good lead comes from complementary therapists, who appear to be particularly effective in this process of helping patients 'to turn the corner'.

If a patient already has a positive attitude to his illness and wants to take action himself then clearly the doctor should encourage this. Sadly, the traditional doctor–patient relationship has tended to stifle such attitudes in patients, and doctors often feel threatened when patients question their treatment or seek out others. At the other extreme, if a patient is not ready to take a positive attitude to his/her disease then simply telling him/her to do so is likely to be counter-productive. It will simply add to his/her list of problems and failures.

It may well be that a successful relationship with a doctor/ healer on a passive level is often a prelude to patients being able to take on a more active healing attitude. This is because one of the effects of a good physician/healer relationship is to improve both self-esteem and confidence. The individual encounter with a good doctor should encourage the patient to find explanations for his/her problems which fit within his/her life story and which enable him/her to take a more active part in looking after his/her health in future. Without any of this, the patient may find it difficult to believe either that he/she is worth healing or that he/she is able to do so him/herself. Thus, within a good therapeutic relationship, the doctor can begin to show the patient how he/she is merely being a catalyst for the self-healing process of the patient him/herself. If the patient begins to take a more positive outlook then the doctor/healer will need to both encourage and guide this progress. In many cases, it may be the positive outlook itself that matters rather than the particular way in which it is channelled. Nevertheless, there are certain ways of channelling this positive outlook and some of these will be discussed briefly in this chapter.

Information/self-help groups

As part of the process of helping a patient to regain his/her sense of control and mastery over his/her illness, it is important that he/she receives as much information as is desirable. In practice, it appears that doctors underestimate the desire of their patients for information in about 65% of encounters.[4] Indeed, one of the best predictors of patient satisfaction is the degree to which the GP provides information.[5] Information alone, however, will not change beliefs, attitudes and behaviour. Our patients require us to give information combined with strategies with which they can respond appropriately to that information.

Information must, therefore, be provided in a way that the patient can understand, remember and use. The communication of a message apparently depends 7% on words, 38% on voice sounds and 55% on body language.[6] Thus, information from the heart may be more useful to some than neutral information, but what matters in the end is only what the patient hears rather than what the doctor says.

Between 37 and 54% of what a doctor tells a patient is forgotten.[7] Not surprisingly then, the listening skills of most people are only 25% effective even though 40% of communication involves active listening.[8] Providing more understandable information and supplying written information have been shown to improve compliance. The importance of proper information has been further highlighted in a recent study on 100 patients with rheumatoid arthritis, where failure to give an adequate explanation of therapy was related to significantly worse perceived pain $(p = .002)$.[9] Patients may also want to know where they can access further information and information on self-help groups and organisations concerned with his/her problem may be very useful. NHS Direct has great potential promise as a source of such information as well.

The word 'doctor' means teacher, but we have failed as teachers if our patients cannot or do not use what we teach them. We have also failed as doctors because they will not improve either.

Relaxation techniques

The importance of stress reduction has been noted several times in this book and its beneficial effects confirmed by work in psychoneuroimmunology. As we have seen, stress may have harmful effects upon the immunological system and coping with stress may both improve immunological status and life expectancy. It may be responsible for a large number of diseases ranging from peptic ulceration and cancer through to coronary artery disease. For instance, social stress has been shown to cause coronary artery disease in monkeys with normal cholesterol levels, while relaxation may improve hypertension, reduce coronary risk and contribute to the reversal of established coronary artery disease.[3,9–12]. As we have seen in earlier chapters, there seems to be good (escapable) and bad (inescapable) stress just as there is good (HDL) and bad (LDL) cholesterol. The highly charged person that is pushing forward the frontiers of his/her life may need no relaxation and the stress may have a positive physical effect upon his/her life. Conversely, a person that is visibly anxious, frustrated and uncomfortable with his/her stress may be helped greatly by anything that promotes even temporary relaxation and relief from anxiety.

There are several options available, which are beyond the scope of this book. Stress reduction groups, meditation, yoga, biofeedback and various forms of exercise offer some treatment pathways. It is of little consequence which system a patient chooses. The important thing is that he/she seeks and finds something that suits him/her.

Positive thinking

Many diseased patients are demoralised patients with negative views of themselves, of others and of anything that may be done to them. Perhaps the main feature of heart sink patients is the negativity that pervades their aura in all those that they meet.

Positive thinking involves the replacement of negative thoughts about the patient with positive thoughts. Valuing one's own importance and worth is a necessary precursor for self-esteem. A positive view of self can then be developed into a positive view of others and life in general.

Matthew Mannings[13] and others have outlined protocols for doing this. For instance, in one exercise the patient is asked to list all the negative beliefs that he/she has about him/herself in one column and all the positive beliefs in another. The aim is to have a comparable number of negative and positive beliefs. After this each negative column is translated into a positive one (e.g. 'I worry too much about other people' becomes e.g. 'I am conscientious'). The objective is for the patient to come to terms with the way he/she is, warts and all, thus become more resistant to disease and better able to cope with it when it occurs.

The sober physician may well fear that this could lead to a nation of 'born again patients'. In reality, it is a slow process where positive reinforcement is essential to alter chronic and ingrained thought processes. Such approaches have proved successful in those patients who are regarded as most untreatable (e.g. this is a central part of the alcoholics anonymous rehabilitation programme). Sometimes the most effective therapists are patients themselves, who have been through this process. They infect those that they meet with that very positivity that they have found for themselves.

Creative visualisation

Creative visualisation is something that patients often instinctively do for themselves. The theory behind creative visualisation is that increasingly coping self-statements and positive images lead in turn to a stronger psychological and physiological resistance to disease. It has been shown, for instance to improve immunocompetence in advanced cancer of the breast.[14]

How is it done? The idea is that the patient should create a visual image of the problem and his/her solution to it. For instance, in cancer therapy an American surgeon encourages his patients to imagine what the tumour looks like, the effects of the treatment given and also to create an image of how their white cells are coping with the problem.[15] The visual imagery is bound to be idiosyncratic because it is personal. One person might visualise white cells as mice eating cheese (the tumour) while another patient may visualise treatment as a row of archers firing arrows at an advancing army (the tumour). The essence of creative visualisation is that the patient should see him/herself as able to exercise some sort of control over the situation. The role of the doctor may be to examine the patient's images in order to confirm that his image of the treatment and the white cells is stronger than the image of the tumour. The patient is also asked to form an image of him/herself fit and healthy and doing all the things that he/she would like to do and this provides a positive aim and direction for recovery.

Self-hypnosis

Any treatment that gets a patient from where he/she is to where he/she would like to be is bound to be beneficial. There are a number of treatments such as neurolinguistic retraining, autogenic regulation and biofeedback, which may be helpful. Self-hypnosis might be seen in some ways as the ultimate weapon in enabling a patient to get his mind and body to do what he wants them to do.

Hypnotherapy, itself, has been shown to improve immunological status, particularly natural killer cells, and reduce episodes of recurrence of genital herpes simplex.[16] Improvement was correlated with reduced levels of anxiety, which may have been the mediating factor. Self-hypnosis in medical students taking examinations was found to reduce the well-documented decline in natural killer cell counts by 45%. Students also felt calmer and had higher energy ratings.

In self-hypnosis, the patient presents structured self-suggestions to him/herself, which have certain characteristics. They should contain a strong desire to get better, be specific with fixed time limits, in simple language, positive and involve exaggeration and emotionalising. Constant repetition of these self-suggestions eventually makes them effective. Patient handbooks are available.[17] Hypnotists frequently help patients to make up their own individualised tapes, which can be used when symptoms recur.

Summary

The end point of any ongoing relationship between doctor and patient should be to put the patient in the driving seat. When it comes to the treatment or prevention of disease, conventional medicine has often done the reverse and made the patient unduly dependent on medical intervention, when it may be inappropriate. Doctors need to be able to nurture their patients as a first step towards them being able to spread their wings and take more active involvement in their own treatment and prevention. A patient who has been through this process may have a powerful influence on others, who have yet to achieve this level of independence. A number of specific approaches are referred to in this chapter but they are not comprehensive and are mentioned only to show the wealth of possibilities that are available. It seems odd in the NHS that the drugs bill should continue to rise at well above the rate of inflation every year, while well-documented treatments such as biofeedback are virtually unobtainable and unheard of. We have not only made our patients dependent we have made society dependent as well. As Fay Weldon puts it: 'The NHS, Oh sacred cow, Oh cruel bitch, has in its forty years produced a very grizzly and unhealthy race of medicine addicted citizens'. The new social, cultural and economic climate should allow this to change. Indeed, the role of the human effect in making patients more actively involved in their own health and welfare will be central if we are to improve public health in the new NHS.

References

1 Wilson A, Hickie I, Lloyd A (1994) Longitudinal study of outcome of chronic fatigue syndrome. *BMJ*. **308**: 756–9.

2 Horwitz RI, Horwirz SM (1993) Adherence to treatment and health outcomes. *Arch Intern Med*. **153**: 1863–8.

3 Ornish D, Brown SE, Scherwitz LW *et al.* (1990) Can lifestyle changes reverse coronary heart disease? *Lancet*. **336**: 129–33.

4 Waitzkin H (1984) Doctor–patient communication. Clinical implications of social scientific research. *JAMA*. **252**: 2441–6.

5 Steptoe A (1991) The links between stress and illness. *J Psychosom Res*. **35** (6): 633–44.

6 Mehrbrabin A (1968) Communication without words. *Psychol Today*. **September**: 53.

7 Ley P (1979) Memory for medical information. *Br J Soc Clin Psychol*. **18**: 245.

8 Burley-Allen M (1982) *Listening: the forgotten skill*. John Wiley, Chichester, UK.

9 Kaplan JR, Manuck SB, Clarkson TB *et al.* (1983) Social stress and

atherosclerosis in normocholesterolemic monkeys. *Science*. **220**: 733–5.

10   Benson H, Rosner BA, Marzetta BR, Klemchuk HM (1974) Decreased blood presure in pharmacologically treated hypertensive patients who regularly elicited the relaxation response. *Lancet*. **i**: 289–91.

11   Patel, C, North WR (1974) Randomised controlled trial of yoga and bio-feedback in management of hypertension. *Lancet*. **ii**: 93–5.

12   Patel C, Marmot MG, Terry DJ *et al.* (1985) Trial of relaxation in reducing coronary risk: four year follow up. *BMJ*. **290**: 1103–6.

13   Mannings, M (1989) *Guide to Self Healing*. Thorson Publishers, Wellingborough, UK.

14   Walker LG *et al.* (1997) Guided imagery and relaxation therapy can modify host defences in women receiving treatment for locally advanced breast cancer. *Br J Surg*. **84** (Suppl.1): 46.

15   Siegel B (1986) *Love and Medicine and Miracles*. Arrow, London.

16   Fox P, Henderson DC, Barton S *et al.* (2000) Immunological markers of frequently recurring genital herpes simplex virex and their response to hypnotherapy. Submitted for publication.

17   Tebbetts C (1990) *Self Hypnosis*. Martin Breese, London.

CHAPTER THIRTEEN

Summary and conclusions

Medicine as we know it is fast moving past the point of no return. Our science, as we currently practise it, is neither sustainable nor fully effective.

In this book we have tried to do just three things. First, to explain the theoretical and ideological void in which we find ourselves and which calls for a new approach. Modern medicine is founded upon a faulty philosophical premise that isolates body and mind, and therefore leaves the patient out of the equation. That is why clinical medicine so often misses the point in what is actually happening between real patients and real doctors. This has led us to emphasise the need for a new approach using what we have called 'the human effect'. We envisage that in future this will lie at the centre of medicine, assisted by clinical evidence, rather than vice versa as has been the dogma of recent years.

Secondly, we have demonstrated the overwhelming evidence on the power of the human effect together with psychoneuro-immunological research, which explains that power. The 'human effect' is by far the most comprehensive and proven treatment that we have – its existence being shown by almost every double-blind placebo-controlled trial. Indeed it is assumed 'a priori' because we have double-blind placebo-controlled trials in the first place. Although we knew about it long before we knew about the proven good effects of streptokinase or aspirin in heart disease, we have largely ignored it. Clinical egos and the clever marketing of medical products may have been part of this. A larger part may also have been self-deception on the part of ourselves as clinicians. We undoubtedly see it least, where it is at its most effective – in young adults of stable temperament with organic disease. In some ways this is a good thing as the human/placebo/healing effect is always at its greatest when both physician and patient believe in the treatment (i.e. there is a folie à deux). It is likely, for instance, that our patients with sore throats and minor upper respiratory tract infections did get better with the antibiotics that we gave them and did improve sooner than they would if we had not given them anything. It is only now that we know that this was not due to any intrinsic action of the antibiotic itself.

Thirdly, we have looked at how we can put the 'human effect' into practice and refine our skills in its use so as to maximise our success as therapists. Part Three of this book is no more than a beginning. Hopefully, it may be the starting point for further books, research and teaching programmes, which will explore in more detail how human beings can maximise their ability to make each other better with or without the use of external chemicals and procedures.

For doctors, this will mean nothing short of a major rethink of our commitment to practice. A rethink of the skills needed for the hugely complex consultations in which we participate daily. A review of the fundamental philosophy which we bring to the privileged work of doctoring. We have to move beyond the metaphor of the body as a machine in our daily work; we need a model that allows us to recognise the importance of our own and the patient's feelings, and the relationships which those feelings construct. If we are arguing to replace Cartesian dualism in medicine, we must also recognise that there is another duality, that of the human person both as object and subject. This allows us to reflect on the important duality that incorporates the externalisation of illness as a disease and the integration of an illness story into the unique context of a person's life. Stories, thus become the central currency of doctoring. Listening to stories, interpreting them, recognising when to 'extract'' from them sufficient material to constitute a disease, and take lead responsibility for defining that; and alternatively emphasising integration of the narrative within the context of the person's life. It is when we emphasise context that we can make use of the skills outlined in this book for the patient's benefit.

Peter Toon, a London GP, has argued for this style of approach in what he terms 'the virtue ethic' of medical practice.[1] Virtues, Toon explains, are constructs which we use to explain, describe or analyse human behaviour; he takes the definition of St Thomas Aquinas as his guide 'The habit or disposition of acting rightly according to right reason'. What this tells us is that the practice of virtue requires not only the intellectual understanding of 'what is right', but the personal attributes required to do the right thing – thus the requirements become attributes of the person, in this case the doctor, not just of the action. Taking an impeccable academic line in tracing the origin and evolution of virtue ethics as a school of philosophy, Toon argues that medical practice can and should be predicated upon the virtues as categorised in western Christian tradition (not because of their intrinsic Christianity, but because the classification is embedded in traditional secular moral thinking). Thus, he argues constructs like fortitude, faith, temperance, charity and hope become central to medical practice. The virtuous practitioner will require both physical and moral courage; the prudence or practical wisdom to exercise sound medical judgement (and thus embrace the benefits of biomechanical science for the patient's good); the temperance, both personal and professional, to support the continuation of consistently virtuous practice; the faith to engage trustingly with patients, to be faithful as it were to them; and to maintain hope in the face of circumstances which tempt us to despair.

These virtues will in their turn encourage the practitioner to act with compassion (to believe from the patient's perspective), to act with humility (setting aside the doctor's own preoccupations to concentrate on the patient's needs to the exclusion of all else) and with responsibility (to embrace the precepts of biomedicine where they apply). Indeed, the virtuous approach to clinical care can be seen as the springboard for much that has been written in the preceding pages.

This book, perhaps, should have carried a health warning for the reader. If these concepts are new to you or if they have any resonance with thoughts that may have been lurking in the back of your mind then you may be about to undergo a permanent change. Analysing, understanding and trying to use the 'human effect' in everyday practice is completely absorbing and is likely to change your perspective on everything that you see and do.

On the plus side, not only will some of your patients start to get better, but your relationships with them will begin to improve and your work should become more challenging and enjoyable rather than yet another effort of drudgery to face the enemy. The inspiring positivism of the human effect leads to a cascade phenomenon in the doctor quite similar to the cascade effect illustrated earlier in this book when trying to explain its action in improving the patient. For the practitioner of the human effect, the range of the possible is ever expanding and few things are impossible. You will know that you have got the bug, when you offer to take on the heart sink patients of your partners and actually relish the prospect and challenge.

The 'human effect' changes doctors. It also changes patients. Those who have fully experienced and understood it will enjoy health benefits far beyond the original symptom or disease for which they saw their doctor. They will be able to hand on this benefit to all those around them. Clearly they cannot be doctors but an effect as powerful as this can be usefully employed by many lay men or women – witness the therapeutic success of many complementary therapies, whose credibility is not accepted by orthodox medicine. In this way it could just be possible to reverse the breakdown in doctor–patient relationships that are blamed on an increasingly demanding and consumerist culture not to mention the increasing problem of litigation.

Consumers are individuals, who go out to get products for themselves. An understanding of the 'human effect' should make it clear to each patient that the product is health and its success is largely a part of themselves and their own self-healing effect. In a culture where the human effect becomes an everyday part of not only the medical consultation, but also of many interactions in the community there will be multiple spin-offs. The patient might cease to be the individual consumer seeking his share of the cake and become an 'NHS citizen' with roles and responsibilities. One who sees his/her role in health disease within the context of all those around. Doctors and patients will need to change in tandem. If PCGs can achieve this end, aided and abetted by doctors, nurses and patients who are committed practitioners of the 'human effect', then the NHS could become the envy of the world. Especially if we can conserve those scarce resources that we need for technological and specialised medicine for where they are absolutely needed. All this calls for a revival of social ideas such as service ethic, social responsibility, social capital and indeed society itself.

Ideals are fine but how do we make them real? First of all we need evidence and this whole neglected area of research needs to be pursued with vigour. We need to know more about what diseases can be helped by the 'human effect' and which can be cured. We need to know more about how to make the 'human effect' maximally effective and more about which aspects, in which situations, in which patients are appropriate for given outcomes. We need to know much more about psychoneuroimmunology – under what conditions can the human effect mimic biologically the provision of external drugs or procedures and whether we can measure this. Perhaps one day we will be able to do a blood test to assess the success of any evidence-based application of 'the human effect' and decide as to whether additional drug therapy is required. This research will be necessary not only to guide our therapy, but also to persuade the sceptics and provide them with the sort of specific evidence base that they require and which frankly does not exist at present. Much of this research will need to be done 'in the field' and PCGs may well provide the ideal context with grounded research that can put therapeutic consultations, health-related services and the local population all under the microscope.[2]

With research and evidence, education and training can follow. It may not be that long before therapeutic competence using the 'human effect' will become as important a part of medical training and assessment as the therapeutic use of drugs and procedures. As we enter the twenty-first century and this book goes to press, this view is partly supported by no lesser a body than the NHS Research and Development Health Technology Assessment Programme.[3] The authors confined their research to the role of expectancy in the placebo effect and concluded that: 'The evidence justifies the training of patients and practitioners in techniques that facilitate patient participation consultations . . . and the training of healthcare professionals may need to be extended to include skills in creating the relevant expectancies in their interactions with patients'. These comments from the orthodox medical establishment represent an important beginning.

New medicine, new values, new vision. It all sounds like the rhetoric of the new NHS. Rhetoric that sometimes appears to use the concept of evidence when it serves its ends, and can seem happy to dump it when political expediency demands it. The 'human effect' is different because it is timeless. What is new is the wealth of recent evidence on its existence and importance at a time when it has become neglected and under-valued. What is called for is less of a revolution and more of a revival. Clinical standards will always be important and the new clinical governance agenda will accelerate their improvement. Much of this improvement, however, will not require the therapeutic or clinical skills of the clinician. For instance, ensuring that patients who have had a heart attack are on aspirin or that they have cholesterol levels that are lower than a certain standard require good organisation, information technology and a key worker, who does not need to be a doctor. Our crucial *clinical* role will remain as diagnosticians while our crucial *therapeutic* role will develop as practitioners of the 'human effect' aided and abetted by medicines and procedures as well as specialist doctors and nurses.

Many are saying that the days of the GP are numbered. If we turn our backs on the 'human effect' then this prophesy will undoubtedly come true. To be both a successful diagnostician in general practice and an effective practitioner of the human effect require high levels of intelligence, expertise and application. Indeed, they present the most difficult, interesting and challenging areas in the whole of medicine. If GPs of the future can do these well, then they will survive. Partly because they will be giving their patients what they need and have consistently asked for. Something that cannot be provided cost effectively by any other means. Partly too because they will have fulfilled the human and social contract that underlied their decision to become GPs in the first place.

References

1   Toon P (1999) *Towards a Philosophy of General Practice: a study of the virtuous practitioner.* Royal College of General Practitioners, London.

2   Kernick D, Stead J, Dixon, M (1999) Moving the reasearch agenda to where it matters. *BMJ.* **319**: 206–7.

3   Crow R, Gage H, Hampson S *et al.* (1999) The role of expectancies in the placebo effect and their use in the delivery of health care: a systematic review. *Health Technol Assess.* **3** (3): 1–38.

Index